Anticancer Herbal Drugs of India

With Special Reference to Ayurveda

Indian Medical Science Series No.124

Anticancer Herbal Drugs of India

With Special Reference to Ayurveda

DR. GYANENDRA PANDEY

Sri Satguru Publications
A Division of
Indian Books Centre
Delhi, India

Published by
Sri Satguru Publications,
Indological and Oriental Publishers
A Division of
Indian Books Centre
40/5, Shakti Nagar,
Delhi-110007
India

Email: ibcindia@vsnl.com
Website: http://www.indianbookscentre.com

First Edition : Delhi 2002

ISBN 81-7030-722-8

Printed at Chawla Offset Printers, Delhi 110 052

Contents

PREAMBLE

Series of investigations have been conducted on cancer by carrying out multi-angled studies with inter-disciplinary approaches in order to find out perfect remedy for this most dreadful disease. Scientific researches in medical sciences are devoting their attention towards various aspects and many kinds of cancer.

The growing popularity of Ayurveda in world traditional systems of medicine is supposed to make delivery in preservance or preventive and remedial or curative aspects of cancer having resemblace with clinical entity of Arbuda in Suśruta Saṁhitā and other compendia followed by various works devoted to indigenous medicine.

Large number of drugs from botanical, mineral and animal sources are employed in treatment of this disease and allied ailing conditions. Survey has been made of such drugs which are mostly from plant origin as herbal therapy is gaining significance in management of cancer.

Review of anti-cancer drugs from sources of indigenous system has been carried out. Observations have been drawn on drug potentials and their inputs towards remedical measures against cancerous conditions. there are majority of three types of drugs : firstly, the drugs recorded and prescribed in classical texts; secondly, the drugs investigated through experiments and studies; and thirdly, the drugs belonging to ethnobotanicals as reported from field survey and tribal medicine. These indigenous drugs open vast avenue of multidisciplinary work.

ROLE OF INDIGENOUS DRUGS AGAINST CANCER (Pandey, G., Abstract of papers, p.29) :

First National conference on Use of Indigenous Drugs in the Management of Cancer (3rd-6th. February, 1988), Faculty of Ayurveda, Institute of Medical Science, Banaras Hindu University, Varanasi, U.P. India.

PROJECT

Present work is preliminary feeuback in the form of a humble, painstaking and scientific attempt to record, collate and review the information on indigenous drugs specifically herbal drugs of India with special reference to Āyurveda, the ancient medical science of Indian School, in the area of oncology, with an object of highlighting anticancer drugs ofplant origins in particular which are evidently supportive to Indian medicine possessing its potentialities-in the terms of clinical concept and drugs efficacy-emerging to fight against cancer, through experiment, assessment, multiangled studies and therapeusis, for better and possible management under cancerology.

DR. GYANENDRA PANDEY

SECTION - I

CANCEROLOGY - ONCOLOGY

(A) Cancer is a malignant growth, formed by the abnormal rapid reproduction of cells. Cancerous cells invasiveness particular properties. The first known as invasiveness, is the capacity to infiltrate and destroy adjacent organs. For example, a cancer of the bowel may spread into the bladder. The second is the ability to form secondary deposits in distant parts of the body. Cancer cells break off from the parent growth and are carried usually in the blood stream to another organs, where they begin to reproduce and form additional tumour masses.

It is not entirely clear whey cancers occur. they principally affects two age groups childrens, and to a much greater extent, people over the age about 40. At present it is believed that cancerous growth in children are related to some form of developmental abnormality, and it is certain that chronic irritation is involved in the later development of cancer.

Treatment for cancer is often effective if the condition is brought to medical attention at an early state. Surgery, X-rays, radium and more recently chemotherapy are commonly used methods and often promote cell recovery.

Patient should consult expert at once if anyone has any of the following symptoms : any unusual lump, bleeding or ulcer, any sudden change in bowel habit, any cough which persists after three weeks, any passing of black motions and unexplained severe weight loss.

Basically and actually, càncer is a malignant tumor of the epithelia! origin. It is specifically hyperplasua of epithelial or gland cell, with infiltration and destruction of tissues.

Etiology of cancer initially finds origin unknown; it may be caused by various forms of chromic irritation. symptomology mainly characterizes some salient and common signs and symptoms viz. persistent discharge from a core that does not heal, discharge from a bleeding from the nipples, blood in the stools or urine or blood-tinged vaginal discharge, persistent pain in the part, a lump esp. in the breast, change in wart or moles, loss of weight, persisent cough or hoarseness.

As regards treatment, the surgery, radium and x-rays are the only recognised effective methods of treatment of cancer. Refrigeration in cases of advanced malignant metastases was in under experimental stage, for alleviation of certain symptoms temporary and improvement of general state of the patient and histological changes in the primary and secondary carcinomatous growth. Various measures, drugs and diets for caring, teating and dealing with normal state and emergencies are recommended under management of cancer which a wide field with varying aspects relevant to kinds, stage and severity of the group of cancer and their complaints.

Most important is early diagnosis and application of proper method or combination of methods are necessary for complete cure Proper, dependable and completely curative therapy for cancer is one of the major subjects of research in medical spheres.

(B.) Tumor is a swelling or enlargement and a neoplasm abnormal prominence of a part, not due to inflammation with no physiological function.

Tumor words pertaining to Angiofibroma, Angiolipoma, Agrenta-fibroma, Astroblastoma, Astrocyotoma, Calor, Carcinosarcoma, Celloma, Calloncus, Cemetoma, Cephalematocele, Ceroma, Cholangioma, Chondroangioma, Chondrofilroma, Chondrolipoma, Chondrosarcoma, Chorioadenoma, Chorioangioma and Chylongioma.

Types of Tumors :

Myelid Sarcometa, Giant Celled S: Consist of elements formed chiefly of protoplasm containing 2 more nuclei, up to 20 or even ; with a varying number of round, spindle or mixed cells. Vary in consistence from that of jelly to that of muscle. More frequently occurs on lower jaw, femur, and tibia.

Round Celled Sarcomata: Usually son vascular, rapidly growing, become large and early give rise to metastatle deposits in distant parts and in visceras. Occur in periosteum, bone, lymphasts glands, subcutaneous tissue, testicle, eye, ovary, uterus, lung, kidneys; though may occur wherever fibrous tissue exists.

Glioma: Grown from the connective tissue of nerve centers and its basic substance resembles that structure. Occurs in retina and brain.

Melanotic Sarcoma: In which cells may be either of round or spindle variety. It is the most malignant form.

Spindle-cell Sarcoma: Cells vary much in size, from small oat-shaped cells to greatly elongated bodies with long, fine, tapering extremities. Chiefly in bones.

Endotheliomata: Attack in different forms the testicle, pia mater, pleurs, and peritoneum.

Acinous or spheroidal-celled Carclnoma: (1) Hard, spheroidal-celled (scirrhus or chronic c.). See: scirrhus. (2) Soft, spheroidal celled (encephaloid, or acute c.); resembles brain tissue in appearance and consistency. Occurs in testicle, liver, bladder, kidney, ovary, fundus ocult, more rarely in the breast.

Colloid Carcinoma: Really one of preceding varieties which has undergones mucoid degeneration, and so distended the alveoli they may be seen by naked eye. Occurs in stomach, intestine, omentum, ovary.

Epithelial Carcinoma: (1) The squamous-celled epithellomata which always spring from skin or mucous membranes.or their glands, esp. at junctions of mucous and cutaneous surfaces. They are not encapsulated. Commence as wart-like growth, flattened tubercle, or fissure, ulceration in all these forms setting in early, (2) Cylindrical or columnar-celled. Less common form of carcinoma. Orginates from either the cylindrical surface epithellum of a mucous membrance, or its glands, closely imitating these structures in microscopic appearance. these growths from sedurated. infiltrating masses in the rolls of organs attacked, producing considerable stenosis of lumen, of hollow rucera; as rectum and small intestinal obstruction. Occur in ulterus and intestinal tract. (3) Tumors composed of spiblastic, hypoblastic, and mesoblastic elements.

Warty or Villous Growth (Papilhmata): Resemble in their structure hypertrophied papillae of skin-or mucous membrance. These include condylomata and mucous tubercles. occur about anus and genitals, or in mouth and throat. Warts and warty growths on skin of hands and genitalla, and mucous surface of larynx. Villous growths, bladder, rectum, and larynx.

Teratoma: tumors containing bone, hair, teeth, etc., situated in ovaries or testicles.

T., connective tissue (chondroma). composed of some variety of connective tissue, forming hard, elastic, slowly growing tumors, often nodular or lobulated. occurs on bones, salivary glands, testicle, etc.

T., fatty (lipoma). consists of adipose tissue, Identical with normal fat. Innocent-grows slowly. May reach large size. Adults - do not recur after removal. occur on shoulders, back, nates. Diffuse form, under chin.

T., fibrous (fibroma). consisting of fibrous tissue. May be dense and firm as a tendon, or soft as areola tissue. Innocent - commonly possess distinct capsule. May occur wherever fibrous tissue is found in any of its forms.

T., glandular (adenoma). Innocent growths originate only from preexisting glandular tissue which they imitate. Two forms: Acinous and tubular. Do not infiltrate the connective tissue. Acinous occur in mammae, lip, ovary, testes, prostate, thyroid, parotid, lacrimal gland, cutaneous and sebaceous glands. Tubular, in intestine, esp. in rectum.

T., lymphatic (vessel) (lymphangloma). Lymphatic vessels are subject to dilatations and varicosities of every degree and extent. To such dilatations in general the term lymphangiectasis is applied, but when by their size, confluence and aggregation they form tumors the term lymphangiomata may be substituted. Occurs on inside of thigh, genitals, on. wall of abdomen.

T., mucous (myxomata). Reseamble the whartonian jelly of the umbillical cord and vitreous humor of the eye. Grows slowly; large size; innocent, not returnning if completely removed. Mucoid softening may attack other forms of tumors. Occurs most frequently in nasal cavities, mammary gland, intermuscular spaces, and submucous and subserous spaces.

f., muscular (myomata). Only those of congenital origin are composed of striated muscle elements (rhabdomyoma), but even in these, the bulk of tumor not composed of muscle cells-new growths made up in part of smooth, nonstriated muscle cells. Occurs in uterus and in prostate, in combintion with fibromata.

Classification of Tumors

Benign	**Malignant**
Generally encapsulated (not invastive)	Not encapsulated invasive).
Slow growing.	Rapidly growing.
Do not metastasize:	metastasize.
Do not interfere with health.	Detrimental to health and life.

I. Connective Tissue Tumors

A. Benign :

(a) Fibroma, composed of fibrous tissue.

(b) Chondroma, composed of cartilage.

(c) Osteoma, composed of bone.

(d) Lipoma, composed of fat.

B. Malignant :

Sarcoma, a cellular tumor composed of any connective tissue cells in disorderly arrangement.

II. Muscle Tissue Tumors

Benign:

Myoma, composed of smooth muscle tissue.

III. Epithelial Tumors

A. Benign:

(a) Papilloma, composed of surface epithellum.

(b) Adenoma, composed of glandular epithelium.

B. Malignant :

(a) Epithelioma, composed of squamous epithelial cells in disorderly arrangement.

(b) Carcinoma, composed of glandular epithelial cells in disorderly arrangement.

IV. Endothelial Tumors

A. Benign :

(a) Hemangloma, composed of blood vessels.

(b) Lymphangioma, composed of lymph vessels.

B. Malignant:

Endothelioma, composed of endothelial cells in disorderly arrangement.

V. Pigmented Tumors

A. Benign:

Nevus, a pigmented mole.

B. Malignant:

Melanoma, pigmented tumor derived from moles.

ONCOLOGICAL CONCEPT IN AYURVEDA

Pathogenesis, symptomology and types of Arbuda.

A. गात्र प्रदेशे कवचिदेव दोषाः संभर्ध्दिता मांसमसृक् प्रदूष्य।
वृत्तं स्थिरं मन्दरूजं महान्तमनल्पमूलं चिरवृद्धये पाकम्।।

B. कुर्वन्ति मांसोच्द्वयमत्यगाघं तदर्बुदं शास्त्रविदो विदान्ति।
तञ्जाये तस्य च लक्षणानि ग्रन्थेः समानानि सदा भवन्ति।

Suśruta Saṁhitā,
nidāna. 11-18/19.

C. Raktārbuda

दोषः प्रदुष्टो रूधिरं सिराश्च संकुच्य सपिंड्य ततस्त्व पाकम्
सास्त्रावमुन्नहयति मांसपिण्डं मांसाङरैराचित माशुवृद्धम्।
करोत्यजस्त्रं रूधिर प्रवृत्तिमसाध्यमेतद्रुघिरात्मकं तु।।
रक्तक्षयोपद्रव पीडितत्वात् पाण्डुर्भवेदर्बुद पीडितस्तु।।

Suśruta Saṁhitā,
nidāna. 11-20/21.

D. Māṁsārbuda

मुष्टिप्रहारादिभिरर्दितेऽङे. मांसं प्रदुष्टं जनयेद्धि शोधम्।।
अवेदनं स्निग्धमनन्यवर्णमपाकमश्मोपमम प्रचाल्यम्।
प्रदुष्टमांसस्य नरस्य गाढ़मेतदवेन्मांस परायणस्य।।

Suśruta Saṁhitā,
nidāna. 11-22/23.

Prognosis

A. Soumyārbuda

मांसार्बुदंत्वेत्तदसाध्यमुक्तं आध्येष्वपीमानि तु बर्जयेच्च।
संप्रस्त्रुतं मर्मणि यच्च जातं स्त्रोतःसुवायच्च भवेदचाल्यम्।।

Suśruta Saṃhitā,
nidāna. 11-24

B. Adhyarbuda

यज्जायतेऽनयत् खलु पूर्वजाते ज्ञेयं तदध्यर्बुदमर्बुद ज्ञैः।
यद्द्वनदूजातं युगपत् क्रमाट्वा द्विरर्बुदंतच्च भवेदसाध्यम।।

Non-pustulative (putrefactive) Characterstic - (pākābhavārbudam)

न पाकमायान्ति कफाधिक त्वान्मेदो बहुत्वाच्च विशेषस्तु।
दोषास्थिरत्वाद् ग्रथनाच्च तैषां सर्वाब्रुदान्येव निसर्गहस्तु।।

Suśruta Saṃhitā,
nidāna. 11-26.

रोगाश्चोत्सेधा–सामान्यात् अधिमांसार्बुदादयः।
विशिष्टा नामरूपाभ्यां निर्देश्या शोथ संग्रहे।

Caraka Saṃhitā,
śūtra.18-33

ग्रन्थ्यबुर्दद्वानां तु यतोऽविशेष प्रदेश हेत्वाकृति दोषद्ष्यैः।
ततश्चिकित्सते भिषगर्बुदानि विहान वित् ग्रन्थि चिकित्सातिना।।

Caraka Saṃhitā,
cikitsā. 12.87.

DIAGNOSIS OF ARBUDA : SUŚRUTA SAMHITĀ, NIDĀNA. 11/
TREATMENT OF ARBUDA : SUŚRUTA SAMHITĀ, CIKITAĀ.18/304

A. VĀTAJĀRBUDA

कर्कारूकैवरूिकनारिकेल प्रियाल पञ्चाडुलबीज चूर्णैः।
वातार्बुदं श्रीरघृताम्बुसिद्धैरूष्णैः सतैलैरूपादाहयेत्तु।
कुयच्चि मुल्यान्झुपनाहनानि सिद्धैश्च मांसैरय वेसवारैः।।

Caraka Saṃhitā,
cikitsā. 18-30

स्वेदं विदध्यात् कुशलास्तु नाड्या
श्रृडे.ग रक्त मृदुशो हरेच्च।
वातघ्ननिर्यूह पयोऽम्लभागैः
सिद्धे शताल्यं त्रिवृत् पिवेत्।।

Suśruta Saṁhitā,
cikitsā. 18-31

B. PITTAJARBUDA

स्वेदोपनाहा मृदवस्तु कार्याः
पित्तार्बुदे कार्यविरेचनं च।
विवृष्य चोदुम्बर शाकागोजी–
पत्रैभृश क्षौद्रयुतैः प्रलिम्पेत्।।

Suśruta Saṁhitā,
cikitsā. 18-32

श्लक्ष्णीकृतैः सर्जरसप्रियङ्गु
पत्तङ्ग रोघ्राञ्जन याष्टिकाह्वैः।
विस्त्राव्य आरग्वधगोजि सोमाः
श्यामा च योज्याः कुशलेन लेपे।।

Suśruta Saṁhitā,
cikitsā. 18-33

श्यामा गिरिह्वाञ्जन कीररसेषु
द्राक्षा रसे सप्तलिका रसे च।
धृतं प्रिवेत् कलीतक संप्रसिद्धि
पित्तार्बुदी तज्जठरी च जन्तुः।।

Suśruta Saṁhitā,
cikitsā. 18-34

C. KAPHAJĀRBUDA

शुद्धस्य जन्तोः कफजेऽर्बुदो तु
एक्तऽवसिक्ते तु ततोऽर्बुदं तत्।
द्रव्याणि यान्यूर्ध्वमधश्च दोषान्
हरन्ति तैः कल्ककृतैः प्रदिहयात्।।

Suśruta Saṁhitā,
cikitsā. 18-35

कपोत पारावतविड् विमिश्रैः
सकांस्यनीलैः शुकलाङ्गलाल्यैः।
मूत्रैस्तु काकादनिमूल मिश्रैः
क्षारप्रदिग्वैव बा प्रदिहयात्।।

Suśruta Saṁhitā,
cikitsā. 18-36

निष्पाव पिण्याक कुलत्थ फल्कै–
मंसि प्रगाढ़ैर्दधमस्तुर्युक्तैः।
लेपविदध्यात् कृमयो यथाऽत्र
मूर्च्छन्ति मुञ्चन्त्यथ मक्षिकाश्च।।
अल्पावशिष्टे कृभिमक्षिते च।
लिखेत्ततोऽग्निं विदधति पश्चात्।
यदल्पनूलं त्रपुताम्रसीस–
पट्टैः समावेष्ट्प तदायसेर्वा

Suśruta Saṁhitā,
cikitsā. 18-37-38

क्षाराग्निशस्त्राण्यसकृद्विदध्यात्
प्राणानहिंसन् भिषग् प्रमतः।
आस्फोत जाती करवीर पत्रैः
कषायमिष्टं व्रणशोधन पत्रैः
कषायमिष्टं व्रणशोधनार्थम्।।
शुद्धे च तैलं विदधीत भार्गी
विडङ्पाठा त्रिफला विपक्वम्।
यदृच्छाया चोपूगत्तानि पाकं
पाकक्रमेणोपचरेद्विविज्ञः।।

Suśruta Saṁhitā,
cikitsā. 18-39-40

मांस दोषन रोग MĀṂSADOṢAJA ROGA

श्रृणु मांसार्बुद कोल गल शाल्क शुण्डिकाः।
पूति मांसालजी गल गण्डमालोपिजिह्विकाः।
विद्यान्मांसाश्रयान्।

Caraka Saṁhitā,
s!utra.28

'अधिमांसार्बुदार्शो अधिजिह्वोप कुशगलशुण्डिकालजी मांसा
संधातौष्ठ प्रकोप–गलगण्ड माला प्रभृतयो मांसदोषजा।'

Suśruta Saṁhitā,
s!utra.24

'मांस गण्डार्बुद ग्रन्थि गण्डोरूदर वृद्धिताः
कण्ठा दिष्वधिमांस च।'

Aṣṭāṅga Hṛdaya,
sūtra

'सास्त्रावमुन्नह्यति मांस पिण्डमाशु कराति च वृद्धिम्।'
'अर्बुदो मांसकीलेऽस्त्री पुरूषे दंशकोटिषु महीघर विशेषो च।'

Medinikośa

स्त्रोतांसि रूधिरादीनां वैषभ्याद् विषमगता
रूद्धारोगाय कल्पन्ते पुष्यन्ति न च द्योतवः
तद्वत् स्त्रोतसां प्रकृतिम्हत्वान्नं विकारे रूप सृज्यते।
शरीरेन्दाहित सेवनात्।
तानि दुष्टानि रोगाय विरुद्धानि सुखाय च।
विकारनामकुशलो न जिन्हीयात् कदाचन।
न हि सर्वे विकाराणां नामतोऽस्ति ध्रुवा स्थितिः।।

Caraka Saṁhitā

गहेनपित्तेन कफेन यापि स्क्तेन मांसेन च मेदसा च।
ज्जायते तस्य लक्षणानि ग्रन्थेः समानानि सदा भवन्ति।
ग्रन्थे समानानि वातिक पैत्तिक श्लौष्यिक।।

Bhāvaprakāśa, madhyamakhaṇḍa., 22.

'महत्तुस्त्राान्थितोर्बुदान वस्तु ग्रन्थिर्महान् ग्रान्थितश्च स्तोऽर्बुदं भवेत्।'

Several preparations as apple products are frequently used in addition to the fruits which are much esteemed among fruits in view of high medicinal, nutritive and dietetic potentials.

MANAGEMENT OF CYST-TUMOR (GRANTHI - ARBUDA)

SOME HERBAL DRUGS–CLASSICAL SOURCES

1. DRĀKṢĀ : Vitis vinifera Linn.

'द्राक्षा रसेनेक्षु रसेन वापि चूर्ण पिबेच्चापि हरीतकीनाम्।

Suśruta Saṁhitā, cikitsā. 18-9

Vṛndamādhava, 41-29

The powder of Harītak (fruits of Terminalia chebula may be used orally after mixing it with the juice of grapes, or Drākṣā (Vitis vinifera) or Ikṣu (sugarcane) (Saccharanum officinarum)

2. DANTĪ : Baliospermum montanum Muell-Arg

दन्ती चित्रकमूल त्वक् सौधर्क पयसी गुड़ः।

भल्लातकास्थि कासीसं लेपो मिन्द्याच्छिलामपि।।

The paste prepared with ingredients comprising Danti, root bark of citraka (Plumbago ziylanica), latex of Snuhī (Euphoribia neriifolia), Arka (Calotropis procera), jaggery (guḍa), Bhallataka nuts (Semecarpus anacardium) and Kāsīsa. It is applied over cyst for breaking (or dissolving) it even a stone.

3. MADHŪKA : Madhuca indica J.F. Gmel.

मधूकजम्बवर्जुनवेतसानां त्वग्भिः प्रदेहान वचारयेत।

सशर्करैर्वा तृणशून्य कन्दैर्दिह्याद भीक्ष्णं भुचुलुन्द जैर्वा।।

Suśruta Saṁhitā,

cikitsā. 18-10

The paste prepared of bark of Madh!uka, Jambu (Syzygium cuminī) Arjuna (Terminalia arjuna) and Vetasa (Salix caprea) is presceribed for local application. It is prescribed specifically in condition of pittaja granthi.

4. KETAKĪ : Pandanus odoratissimum Linn.f.

'सशर्करैर्वा कन्दैर्दिंह्याद भीक्ष्णं भुचुलुन्द जैर्वा।'

Suśruta Saṁhitā,

cikitsā. 18-10

The root of Ketakī mixed with sugar (śarkarā) is ground and its paste is applied externally.

5. MUCAKUNDA : Pterospermum ācerifolium Willd.

'सशर्करैर्वा तृणशून्य कन्दैर्दिह्याद भीक्ष्णं मुचलुन्द जैर्वा।'

The flowers of Mucakunda mixed with sugar are ground for making them into a paste which is useful to applied locally.

6. MULAKA : Raphanus sativus Linn.

क. लेपनं शंखचूर्णेन सह भूलकमस्मना।
कफार्बुदापहं कुर्याद् ग्रन्थ्यादिषु विशेषतः।।
Vṛndamādhava, 41-37.

The paste of Śankha (conch-shell) powder or bhasma, mixed with ash of (raddish) is recommended to be applied locally. it is considered to effective specially in Kaphajārbuda (tumour) and grandhi (cyst) and other similar conditions.

7. SAIREYAKA : Barleria prionitis Linn.

'सिराग्रन्थे त्वमिनवे तैलं सहचरं पिवेत्।'
Aṣṭāṅga Sangraha,
Uttara. 35-13.

The oil is prepared with whole plant of Saireyaka or sahacara (by cooking plant material or Kalka in oil under taila pāka process). Saireyaka oil is indicated for application externally in acute stage of sirāgranthi (cyst in blood vessels).

8. ŚAMI : Prosopis cineraria Druce.

शमीमूलक शिग्रूणां बीजैः सयवसर्षवैः।
लेपः पिष्टोऽम्लतक्रेण ग्रन्थिगण्ड विलापनः।।
Aṣṭāṅga Hṛdaya,
uttara. 30-16.

The paste is prepared in combination of the seeds of Śamī, Mulaka (Raphanus sativa), Śigru (Moringa oleifera), barley (yava) and mustard (sarṣpa), with sour better-milk (takra). It is applied locally for disintegrating (vilāpana) cysts granthi and glands (gaṇḍa).

9. SURANA : Amorphophallus campanulatus Blume.

क. परिणत सूरणकन्दे सनागरं तोयसंपिष्टम्।
मेदोग्रन्थिहरार्थं लिम्पेद् बहुशश्च सप्ताहम्।।
Vaidya Manoramā,
16-139.

The mature tuber of Sūraṇa is mixed with ginger powder (śuṇṭhī) and pounded with water for preparing a paste which is applied on the cyst (granthi); Its application is frequently suggested for continuing for a week (or depending on the need)

ख. सौरणं कन्दकं दग्ध्वा घृतेन च गुडेन च।
लेपनञ्चार्बुदानाञ्च नाशनञ्च भिषग्वरः।।
Hāriīta Saṃhitā, 3-37-6.

The tuber of sūraṇa is firstly burnt and then mixed with ghee and jaggery. This paste is applied externally for destroying the tumor (arbuda).

10. SNUHĪ : Euphorba neri folia Linn.

'स्नुही गण्डीरिकास्वेदो नाशयेदर्बुदानि च।'
Vṛnadamādhava, 41-44.

The fomentation of stem-piece of snuhī is prescribed externally for destroying the tumors.

11. ŚYONĀKA : Oxoxylum indicum Vent.

'हिंस्त्रादि योग।'
Suśruta Saṃhitā,
Cikitsā. 18-5.

The drug Śyonāka is an ingredient of the formulation Hiṁsrādi-yoga prescribed in treatment of disease (granthi cyst).

12. UPODIKĀ : Basella rubra Linn.

`क. उपोदकारसाम्यक्तास्तत् पत्र परिवेष्टिताः।
प्रणश्यन्त्य चिरात्रृणां पिटकार्बुदजातयः।।
Vṛndamādhava, 41-42.

The juice of Upodikā is applied to annoint the boils (piṭakā) and tumours (arbuda) and they are covered (pariveṣṭana) with the leaves of upodikā for their pacification.

ख. उपोदका काञ्जिकतक्रपिष्टा तयोपनाहो लवणेन मिश्रः।
दृष्टोऽर्बुदानां प्रशभाय कैश्चिद् दिने दिने रात्रिषु मर्मजानाम्।।
Vṛndamādhava, 41-43.

The plant and leaves are ground with sour gruel and butter milk with salt for preparing a poultice (upanāha) which is applied on tumours (arbuda).

13. VIKANKATA : Flacourtia romantchi L. Herit

विकङ.तारग्वघकाकणन्ती काकादनी तापसवृक्ष मूलैः।
आलेपयेत् पिण्डफलार्क भार्गी करञ्ज काला भदनैश्च विद्वान्।।
Suśruta Saṁhitā,
Cikitsā. 18-13.

The paste of vikankata, Aragvadha and some other drug plants (Kākādanī, Kākaṇantī, tāpasavṛkṣa m!ula etc.) is recommended to apply on cyst specially caused by kapha (kaphajanya granthi).

14. VANYAKĀRPĀSI : Thespesia lampas Dalz.&Gibs.

'उत्तुण्डिकांध्रिरूपलेपनतः स आशु ग्रन्थीन विनाशयति सार्बुदगण्डमालान्।'

Rājamārtaṇḍa, 27-2.

The root of vanyakārpāsī is pounded for making a paste which is applied externally on cyst, tumour and cervical adenitis for their alleviation.

15. ŚIGRU : Moringa oleifera Lam.

शिग्रुम्लकयोर्बीजं रक्षोघ्नं सुरसा यवम्।
तक्रेणाश्वरिपुं पिष्ट्वा लिम्पेदार्बुद शान्तये।।
Bhāvaprakāśa, madhya. 44-57

The paste of seeds of Śigru, M!ulaka, Sarsapa, Indrayava and root of Karavīra is suggested to be prepared with butter milk (takra); is locally applied on arbuda (tumour).

16. VATA : Ficus bengalensis Linn.

वटदुग्ध कुष्ठरोमक लिप्तं वद्धं वटस्य पत्रेण।
अध्यास्थि सप्तरात्रान्महदप्युशन्तिमर्बुदं गच्छेत्।।

Bhāvaprakāśa,
madhya. 44-56.

The latex of vaṭa mixed with kuṣṭha (Saussurea lappa), romaka (sambhar salt) is prescribed for local application on arbuda (tumour). The leaves of vaṭa or nyagrodha are suggested for tying up ('vaddham vaṭasya patreṇa') over tumour (arbuda). It has been indicated (and claimed) that the appliction of vaṭa may pacify arbuda, even very big tumorous growth on bone;(ādhyasthi) within a period of a week.

17. HARIDRĀ : Curcuma domestica Linn.

हरिद्रालोघ्रपत्राङ्ग गृहघूम मनःशिलाः।
मधु प्रगाढ़ो लेपोऽयं मेदोऽर्बुदहरः परः।।

Bhāvaprakāśa, madhya-44-54.

The powder of haridrā in combination with Lodhra, (symplocos racemosa) patrāṅga, house-smoke (grahadhūma) and manḥśilā, is mixed with honey for preparing a paste and the same is recommended to locally apply on tumour specially medajārbuda., as external remedy

तल्लक्षण च मेदान्तेऽषोढ़ा दोषादिभिस्तु तत्।
प्रायो वेद कफाढ्यत्वात् स्थिर त्वाच्च न पच्यते।।

Aṣṭānga Sangraha,
U. 34-3/14-15

'तस्यार्बुदस्य लक्षणं ग्रन्थिपठिते मेदान्तैर्दोषादिभिः षोढ़ा।
अनेनास्थिसिराव्रणजानां प्रतिषेधः।
तच्चार्बुद मेदः कफाद्घत्वात् स्थिरत्वाच्च हेतोः प्रायो न पच्चते।'

4-15

STUDIES ON ANTICANER PLANTS AND DRUGS

Recent researches conducted by a group of chinese scientists working in the Institute of Virology find that some fresh vegetables such as carrots, turnips, gourd and sprous contain interferon-inducer, which stimulā cells to produce interferon, a protein which can increase human resistance to virus infections. Interferon-inducer can therefore be effective against caner.

A report of I.C.M.R. (Indian Council of Medical Research) from India finds the number of patients in India affected by cancer of mouth and ocsaphagus in the year 1986 was 56000 and till 2001 they will be increasing to 86000. Similarly the number of lung cancer cases will be increased from 27000 to 40000. till todate a very limited number of plant products are used for treatment of cancer and the investigations of plants for finding out remedies against cancer are also limited specially from the vast group of indigenous drugs.

Cancer is one of the most dreaded diseases of the 20th century and spreading further with continuance and increasing incidence in current 21st century, plagning the life of mankind. It is considered a negative and adversary of modernisation and advanced pattern of socio-cultural life dominated by westernisation Modern medicine and multi-disciplinary scientific investigations are making best efforts for combating the disease, but the sure-shot, perfectly curative and fully suitable cure is yet to be brought out in world medicine.

Since the Cancer is a global problem of serious nature and the concerted and active efforts of medical and bioscientists including chemists have got success and several enticancer remedies of synthetics and natural both.

Several of modern drugs, foods and other edible articles have carcinogenic effects on human. Various anti-cancer medicines and therapies applied for may clinical management of several kinds of cancer and malignancy conditions result more or less severe side-effects and problematic complications in cancer patients. Moreover, the drugs, therapies and proper cancer treatment (including under/ socio-psychological conditions patient care) are tidious, costly and sometimes discouraging or hopeless, little optimism for complete and steady recovery.

Recently, the greater emphasis has been given towards the researches on plants products and drugs from botanical origins for investigating anti-tumor and anti-cancer efficacy of medicinal plants in order to detect evaluate and select the anticancer herbal agent. natural as cure of diseases. The primitive people were acquainted withs the plant remedies in addition to be sure of plant knowledge preserved in ancient medical texts. Series of studies have been condicted on folklores under ethnobotanical researches. For the instance,J.Hartwell L (Loydia, 1967-71) has collected data on about 3,000 plants which possess anticancer properties and various drug plants belonging to this kind of investigatory plan projects have later became potential anti-cancer drugs and effective remedies of other diseases.

Diets, Vegetables and Phytochemicals-Cancer Risk and Prevention

The American scientific efforts in the field of oncology also remarkably include the activities of the National Cancer Institute in America, for launching a multimillion dollar project to find, isolate and study the phytochemicals in vegetables of importance belonging to vitamins plant origin (Bagley, Sharon, Beyond Vitamins, Newsweek, April 25, 1994.) Since the research on phytochemicals in vegetables, other than plants in general, a large battery of chemicals from caulifollowers to pineapples and from muringa shoot to red chillies are now has been found and they are under active investigations. These chemical originally evolved to protect plants from seenlight have gained basic and prime importance in controlling cancer in human beings.

I. Vegetables Protecting Cancer

Amazing tongue-twisters these quaintly phrased phytochemicals have such an enormous range of activities, that it has marked an explosive beginning of the anticancer crusade. In fact, all fruits and vegetables contain these powerful cancer-fighting phyto-chemicals, which reveals the wisdom of our ancestors in recommending a vegetarian diet full of fruits and vegetables. And our foolishness for discarding it for fast food, processed food and multivitamin tablets of various hues, which are all poor substitutes for whole foods especially fruits and vegetables. According the Bagley, they harbour a whole ratatouille of compounds that have never seen the inside of a vitamin bottle for the simple reason that scientists have not, until very recently even known they existed, let along brewed them into pills. Some of the phytochemicals isolated and their functions are given in table containing selelected vegetables.

Defusing of tumours :

Right now everybody is confused about many long-accepted tenets of nutrition. For instance the role of cholesterol in heart disease, the place of coconut oil in dietetics, the question of first class and second class proteins are all being hotly contested. perhaps the most crippling of the blows was the doubt cast on the ability of antioxidant vitamins like Betacarotene and vitamin C in preventing cancer., which was hailed as a great modern discovery. According to Dr. Julie Buring of boston, USA, āmong all the substances, phytochemicals offer the next great hope for the magic pill, one that would go beyond vitamins.

Kicking out the carcinogen

The most promising of the phytochemicals is perhaps SULFORAPHANE found in broccoli, cauliflower, brussels sprout, turnips and kale. The fact that cooking or microwaving the vegetables does not destroy it enhances its value. In 1992, Dr. Paul Talalay of Johns Hopkins Medical College, Baltimore, USA added Sulforaphane to human cells growing in tissue culture and showed that it boosted synthesis of anticancer enzymes. Later he took 3 groups of rats and injected them with DMBA, a known carcinogen. while the first group served as controls, the second set was injected with low doses and the third group with high doses of Sulforaphane. Surprisingly while 68% of the rats in Group I got mammary tumours, in the second group only 35% and in the third only 26% developed these tumours. Prof. Gary Posner, of the chemistry department of the same institute produced Sulforaphane synthetically. When this synthetic material was injected into a fourth of set of rats, the results were even more fantastic. Only 25% of the rats developed cancer.

It seems that sulforaphane works its magic by snuffing out the cancer before it begins. The first step in the production of cancer begins. the first step in the production of cancer begins with a cancer-producing i.e. Carcinogen molecule from food, drink, air of smoke invading cell. Within hours after being eaten, sulforaphane enters the blood stream and reaches the cell and stimulates a grup of proteins called phase II enzymes. The enzymes burst into action, attaching the Carcinogen to a molecule that kicks it out of the cell.

	Name of the vegetables	Name of the phytochemicals	Functions of the phytochemicals
1.	Cauliflower (broccole)	Sulforaphane	Sets in motion a process that whisks Carcinogens out of cells.
2.	Do	PEITC binding to DNA.	Prevents Carcinogens from binding to DNA.
3.	Do	Indole-3-Carbinol	Helps a precursor of the hormone oestrongen, break up into a benign rather than a cancer causing form.
4.	Citrus fruits and berries	Flavenoids	Prevents cancer-causing hormones from hatching on to a cell.
5.	Tomatoes, green chillies, pineapple and strawberries	P. coumaric Acid	Disrupts and the chemicals combination between two common molecules which detoxify carcinogens.
6.	Garlic and onions	Allylic Sulfides	Protects against stomach cancer. They stimulate intracellular enzymes which detoxify carcinogens
7.	Soya	Genistein	Prevents tiny tumours from getting connected to the capillaries that carry oxygen and nutrition killing the tumour cells.
8.	Red chilly	Capsaicin	Prevents carcinogens like those in cigarette smoke from binding to DNA, where they can trigger lung cancer.

Multiple blockages :

Researches done in the last two decades have convinced scientists that the production of cancer is by a complicated multifaceted chemical protocol. In fact theoretically it is impossible to have Cancer, as a cell has to pass through so many biochemical loops before it can become cancerous. In spite of all this, more than 2% of the world's population do get cancer. the multiplicity of the steps in the production of cancer is at once an insoluble problem for the seeker of the aetiology of cancer, while for the researcher trying to block cance,r it is a godsend. Fortunately, as it turns out, one or more of the inumerable compounds found in vegetables are capable of blocking the process at one stage or another.

During the process of digestion, our body routinely makes compounds, called nitrosamines out of nitric acid and anines derived from proteins. production of nitrosamines are the first step in carcinogenesis. Tomato has nearly 10,000 phytochemicals in it. of these, two i.e. P. coumaric acid and Chlorogenic acid catch hold of the nitric acid and whisk it out of the cell before its combination with amines. When Prof. Hotchkiss of Cornell University of USA have tomato juice to volunteers, their bodies made fewer nitrosamines. According to him, the whole tomato is more effective than the vitamin component. One can't have a lousy diet and take a few vitamins and get the same benefit. It is heartening that these acids are seen in many fruits and vegetables including green chillies, pineapples, strawberries and carrots.

The kaleidoscope of vegetable chemicals:

As shown in the table, almost every vegetable in loaded with phytochemicals, thousands fo them as for example in tomatoes. cabbages and cauliflowers (for as Mark Twain put it, what is a cauliflower after all, but a cabbage with college education?) have it. Green chillies, red chillies, tumeric, cumin are all loaded with it. and almost every fruit and vegetable from berries to yams, to citrus and cucumbers contains flavinoids. To quote Bagley "In a cellular version of musical chairs, these compounds race to sites on the cell, where cancer-causing hormones attach themselves. When the music stops, they keep the hormones from sitting down on the cells' surface."

The research work, as is obvious has been confined to USA and Europe. hence only vegetables and fruits found in the temperate climate have been subjected to scientific scrutiny. the tropical areas have a kaleidoscopic variety of fruits and vegetables, and the biological diversity of this areas is incomparable. so it only stands to reason that thousands, may millions of phytochemicals can be found in the tropical fruits and vegetables, if planned research work is undertaken. Vegetables and fruits like bannas, yam, gooseberry, mangoes, guava, melons, tamarind, jackfruit An anticancerous lectin has been identified in Jackfruit which has been used as home remedies for various chronic diseases in our country from days of yore are sure to be gold mines of phytochemicals. So also leaves and shoots of muringa, different verieties of Keerai, neem, karuveppila, Pudina and others. A co-ordinated approach in this area with the combined efforts of modern doctors, Ayurvedic physicians, ethanobotanists, pharmacologists, chemists and biologists will yield fantastically rich dividend (Vegetables against Cancer, Kutty, K.M.,Arya vaidyan, Vol.8, No. 1 August, pp.14-27). Thus, the diet, vegetables recommended in Indian way of life and Indian Medicine find strong scientific support in the area of cancer for its control.

II. Diet and Basal Cell Carcinoma of the Skin in a Prospective Cohort of Men.

Nonmelanoma skin cancer is the most common form of malignancy in white populations. The two primary histologic types of nonmelanoma skin cancer are basal cell carcinoma (BCC) and squamous cell acids hve been associated with increased squamous cell carcinogenesis. the Health Professionals Follow-up Study started in 1986 when 51529 male health professionals completed a questionnaire on medical history and known and suspected risk factors for cancer and other major illnesses.

A detailed description of the 131-item semiquantitative food-frequency questionnaire used in this study and decumentation of its reproducibility and validity have been published. Briefly, for each food, a commonly used unit or portion size was specified and participants were asked to indicate for each food how often, on average, they had consumed the amount specified during the past year. also the type of breakfast cereal eaten; the brand, dose, duration and frequency of multivitamin use; the dose and duration of use of individual vitamin supplements; and the types of fat commonly used for cooking and at the table were enquired. The nutrient intakes were computed by multiplying the consumption frequency of each unit of food by the nutrient content in the specified portion. the values for the nutrient amounts in foods were obtained from the Harvard University Food Compsosition Database.

During 308071 person-years of follow-up from 1986 through 1994, 3190 incident cases of BCC were reported. Higher total fat intake was associated with a lower risk of BCC. When saturated fat, monounsaturated fat (predominantly oleic acid), polyunsaturated fat (predominantly linoleic acid), and long-chain n-3 fatty acids were included in the multivariate model simultaneously, only monounsaturated fat (Relative risk (RR) for highest quintile: 0.79; 95% CI: 0.65, 0.96) and long-chain n-3 fatty acids (BR: 1.13; 95% CI: 1.01, 1.27) were significantly associated wityh BCc risk. Including dietary cholesterol, trans fatty acids, or folate in the multivariate models carcinoma. Basal cell carcinoma in men is about 4 times as common as squamous cell carcinoma. Metastatic spread of BCC is rare, but the malignancy is associated with substantial morbidity and high health-care cost. Although sun exposure is the main established risk factor for BCC, diet also influences the development of BCC.

Higher intake of total fat, and lower intakes of beta-carotene, retinol, vitamin E, vitamin C, vitamin D, and long-chain n-3 fatty with monounsaturated fat did not appreciably change the results. Furthermore, a highly significant negative trend with higher intakes of monounsaturated fat were observed across deciles of intake (multivariate RR: 0.76; 95%) intake of retinol, folate, vitamin C, and vitamin D were positively associated with risk of BCC.

When retinol, carotene, folate, vitamin C, vitamin D, and vitamin E were included simultaneously in the multivariate model, only folate and vitamin C remained associated with BCC risk remained significant after adjustment for monounsaturated or total fat. Consumption of vegetables was not significantly associated with BCc risk. The intake of folate and vitamin D tended to be positively associated with thr risk of BCC. However, the tests for trend were not significant. Carotene intake was significantly associated with the risk of BCc. This inverse association was due to an association of alpha-carotene and beta-carotene with risk of BCC.

The findings do not support the hypotheses that low intake of fat or high intakes of long-chain n-3 fatty acids, retinol, carotene, folate, or the vitamins C,D,or E decrease the risk of BCC. By contrast, high intake of monounsaturated fat and low intake of folate were associated with a swmall decrease in BCc risk. in general, nutrient intakes assessed by the questionnaire were strongly correlated with the estimates from diet records.

A 20% higher risk of BCC for the third quintile of folate intake (median; 388 ug/d) as compared with the lowest quintile was observed; higher intake did not further increase BCC risk. Also there was no protective effect for retinol, carotene, or vitamins C,D, or E. Basal cell carcinoma risk was not significantly associated with serum concentrations of retinol, beta-carotene, lycompene, alpha-tocopherol or dietary vitamin A.

An inverse association between monounsaturated fat consumption and BCC risk was observed. Saturated and polyunsaturated fat were not associated with BCC risk after adjustment for monounsaturated fat intake. Also no increase in risk of BCc in participants with high fat intakes was observed. However, our results do not suggest that a diet low in fat or high in specific nutrient substantially reduces risk of BCC in men during an 8-year period (Van Dam, R.M. et al, Fm. J. clin, Nutr., 2000, 11, 135. Abstract in Probe, Vol. 34, No. 4, July-Sept., 2000, pp. 298-300).

ANTI-OXIDANTS AGAINST CANCER - VEGETABLES FRUITS AND HERBS

The starting point of some of the scariest diseases known to man, the cell. Cancer, Heart diseases, diabetes mellitus, Arthritis. They all begin of the cell. They have a common name, degenerative or one-related diseases, and the process that cause them is going on inside your body. Now the main causes of degenerative diseases is damage to healthy cells, mostly by oxidation.

What is oxidation. Have you ever seen the cut portion of an apple turn down. This reaction is called oxidation. it is also the process that your body every time you breath. But the downside is that cogue molecules called free radicals can oxidise healthy cells, starting an oxidation chain reaction. One damaged cell produces more free radicals, which damage more cells which lead to tissue damage, and finally disease

Are you at risk. Our diet and life styles have changed. Loss of food comes from fresh sources (that help prevent oxidation damage), noticed how we eat more refined and packaged foods.

Also, free radicals production is stepped or by exposure to air pollution, increased ultra-violet radiation, due to zone layer depletion, and contaminants in foods and water. Smoking, lack of sleep, unplanned diets and physical and mental stress also increase oxidation damage; and therefore the risk of degenerative diseases.

Can oxidation damage be stopped. No, but it can be reduced dramatically. You can do this by adopting a healthy lifestyle, and you can also make sure you get enough anti-oxidants.

What are anti-oxidants. Anti-oxidants are benefecial compounds that neutralise free radicals before they can attack healthy body cells. Examples of anti-oxidants are vitamin C, Vitamin E, Carotenoids and mineral such as zinc and selenium. They are part of your daily diet fruit and vegetables are major sources. But to get enough, you must add 5 servings of fruits and 5 servings of vegetables.

It is possible to add enough fruits and vegetables everyday. A richest source nature of carotenoids comes from the micro-algae Dunoliella salina. Some other best ani-oxidants among nature are the yellow pigments found in yellow orange, red some green fruits and vegetables (carrot, orange etc.)

Carotene is a safe source of vitamin A (the body converts carotene to vitamin A as and when required). But importantly, it acts as a potent anti-axidants protecting you from the coverage of free radicals damage, reducing the risk of degenerative dixaxs like cancer, diabetes, heart diseases, arthritis, sttress reactions, cataract and other muscular degeneration conditons. (The Hindustan Times, 23-12-2000, Advt. p. 23).

GREEN MAGIC - HERB AGAINST CANCER

While eating vegetables is often touted as a way to fight diseases, excactly, how they promote health is not clear. Now, researchers think they know how the body used at least one vegetable as a weapon against cancer.

Researchers from the University of California at berkeley looked at the effects of brocoli on human breast cancer cells.

According to findings compounds in brocoli known as indoles are digested and broken down in the stomach to a compound celled 3,3 - dindoly - methane (DIM.) This compound may be the key to keeping cancer at bay. DIM prevents malignant cells from dividing and multiplying, thereby preventing the spread of cancer. it also promotes the death of tumour cells by increasing levels of a protein that kills cells and lowering levels of another protein that keeps cells alive. (The Hindustan Times, Fitness 5, 24-12-2000).

APPLE AGAINST CANCER

An Apple a day keeps doctor away is a famous proverb. It is really scientifically true. Apple is highly valued fruit not only for its taste but also for its health promoting qualities.

Apple is known as valuable plant produce as desert fruit which contains vitamins (A,B,C and E), calcium, silica, sodium, sulphur, iron, magnesium chlorine, bromine and other trace elements.

Besides the medical science and various systems of medicine appreciate in general the potentialities of apple comprising preventive and curative properties as health restorative as well as medicine including wholesome food and fruit in a number of diseases. Cancer is one of the important diseases of present day concern for which the apple is widely recommended. In various countries, the apples fruits are given as part of diet of cancer patients for relief. It helps in overcoming such ailments as diarrhoea, loss of appetite, gas problem, weakness resulting from prolonged illness, constipation and particularly heart diseases. it is nutritional fruit as a good general tonic for healthy and diseased persons.

Section II

HERBAL DRUGS USEFUL AGAINST CANCER

	DRUG	SOURCE PANT	HABIT	PARTS USED
1.	Upodikā	Basell eubra L.	Herb	Whole Plant,
2.	Kadalī	Musa sapientum L.	Large shrub	Leaves Root
3.	Śālmalī	Salomalia malabaricum (Dc.) Sch. & Endl.	Tree	Roots, flowers, bark
4.	Yava	Hordeum vulgare L.	Grass, cereal	Seeds-(grains); yawakṣāra
5.	Viḍaṅga	Embelia ribes (Burm.)f.	Shrub or small tree	(alkalies-ash, Seeds)
6.	Kāncanāra	Bauhinia variegata L.	Tree	Bark, flowers
7.	Śuṇthī	Zingiber fficinale Rose.	Herb	Rhizomes-green and dried
8.	Kāncanāra	Bauhimia racemosa Lamk.	Tree, small or medium sized tree	

9.	Śigru	Moriinga oleifera Lam.	small tree or moderate sized tree	ark, leaves, pods
10.	Guggulu	Comniphora wightii (Arun.)	Shrubs	leogum resin
11.	Bhallātaka	Semecarpus ancanrdium Linn.	ee	·uit (nut)
12.	Rohitaka (rakta)	Tecomella undulata (Sm.) eam.	ee	ark
13.	Śākhoṭaka	treblus asper Lour.	ıall or moderate ze tree	ark
14.	Nimba	zadirachta indica Juss.	ee	eaves, inner bark, ark, bark etc.
15.	Madayantikā	Lawsonia inermis L.	ırub	eaves
16.	Cāngerī	Oxalis corniculata L.	erb	/hole Plant
17.	Pāṣāṇabheda	Bergenia ligulata Yes.	erb	oots
18.	Śarapunkhā	Tephrosia purpurea Pers.	erb or under ırub	oots
19.	Amarvallī	Cuscuta reflexa Roxb.	vining herb	lant
20.	Svarṇakṣirī	Agremone mexicana L.	rrickly herb	atex, roots, leaves, seeds
21.	Punarnavā	Boerhaavia diffusa L.	Prostrate herb	oots Leave

22.	Bhṛngarāja	Eclipta prostrata (L.) Linn.	Herb	Whole plant
23.	Manjiṣṭhā	Rubia cordifolia L.	Climber	Roots
24.	Tila	Sesamum orientale L.	Herb or under shrub	Seeds
25.	Drākṣā	Vitis vinifera L.	Climber	Fruits
26.	Kirātatikta	Swertia chirayita (Roxb. ex Flem.) Karsten.	Under shrub	Whole plant, roots
27.	Rāsnā	Pluchea lanceolata C.B. Clarke.	Herb	Roots leaves whole plant.
28.	Muṇḍī	Sphaeranthus indicus L.	Herb	Whole plant, flowers.
29.	Guḍ!ucī	Tinospora cordifolia (L.) Merr.	Climber	Stem.
30.	Harītakī	Terminalia chebula Retz.	Tree	Fruits
31.	Bibhītaka	Terminalia bellirica (Gaertn.)	Roxb. Tree	Fruits
32.	Āmalakī	Emblica officinalis Gaertn.	Tree	Fruits
33.	Karkaṭaśṛṅgī	Pistacia chinensis Bunge. ssp. integerrima (Stew.) Rech.f.	Tree	Follicles
34.	Droṇapuṣpī	Leucas cephalotes (Roth.) Spr.	Herb whole plant	Leaves,

35.	Nirguṇḍī	Vitex negundo L.	Shrub	Roots, leaves, Bark.
36.	Rohitaka (śveta)	Aphanamixis polystachya (Wall.)	Parker Tree	Bark, seeds, leaves.
37.	Fraṇḍa	Ricinus communis L.	Shrub	Roots, seeds, leaves.
38.	Harītakī	Terminalia chebula Retz	Tree	Fruits
39.	Dāruharidrā	Berberis aristata Dc.	Hormy shrub	Root, bark, fruits
40.	Bhūmyāmalakī	Phyllanthus fraternus Webst.	Prostrate herb	Whole plant,
41.	Kāsamarda	Cassia occidentalis Linn.	Tall herb	Various parts
42.	Ariṣṭaka	Sapindus emarginatus Vahl.	Tree	Fruit, bark
43.	Ahiphena-phala	Papaver sonniferum L.	Under shrub	Fruit (poppy)
44.	Eraṇḍakarkaṭī	Carica papaya L.	Shrub	Fruits, latesc
45.	Brāhmī	Bacopa minnieri (L.) Penn.	Herb	Whole plant
46.	Maṇḍ!ukaparṇī	Centella asiatica (L.)	Urban.	Herb, prosprate whole plant
47.	Babbūla	Acacia nilotica (L.) Del. ssp. indica (benth.) Bren.	Thorny tree	Bark, pods, gum.
48.	Punarnavā Varṣābhū	Boerhaavia chinensis (L.) Asch. & Schw.	Prostrate herb	Roots

49.	Sadāpuspī	Catharanthus roseus (L.) Don	Herb	Whole plant. leaves.
50.	Ratnajyoti (Ratenjot)	Arnebia benthami (Don.) John. syn. Macrotomia benthami DC.		Roots
51.	Illar-villar	Cocculum pendulus (JR.&G.) Forst.		Leaves
52.	Gidar tamaku	Verbascum thapsus L.	Herb	Leaves
53.	Garjarapatrikā	Parthenium hysterophorous L.	Herb. weed	Leaves, whole plant
54.	Khadira	Acacia catechu (L.f.) Willd.	Thorny tree	Bark, heart-wood
55.	Gojihvā	Onosma bracteatum Wall.	Herb	Roots
56.	Trivṛtt	Operculina turpethum (Linn.) Silva Manso	Twining plant	Roots
57.	Priyangu-puṣpa priyangu	Callicarpa macrophylla Vahl.	Under shrub	Flowers. Fruits
58.	Pattanga	Caesalpinia sappan Linn.	Small tree	Heart word.
59.	Akṣoṭa	Juglans regia L.	Tree	Bark. tree
60.	Udumbara	Ficus racemosa L.	Tree	Bark. frui

61.	Lodhra	Ficus glomerata Roxb.	Tree	Bark
62.	Ingudī	Balanites aegyptiaca (Linn.) Delile.	Small tree	Fruit, seeds.
63.	Lāngalī	Gloriosa superba L.	Herb	Rhizomes
64.	Puṣkaram!ula	Inula racemosa Hook.f.	Herb	Root
65.	Kulatthikā	Macrotyloma uniflorum (Lamk.) Verd.	Herb, cereal	Seeds (Pulse)
66.	Sārivā	Cryptolepis buchanani Roem & Schutt.	Climber	Roots, latex
67.	Vāsā	Adhatoda vasica Nees.	Shrub	Leaves, flowers, roots
68.	Mustaka	Cyperus rotundus L.	Herb	Rhizomes
69.	Candana-rakta	Pterocarpus santalinus Linn.	Tree	Heart-wood
70.	Bilva	Aegle marmelos Corr.	Tree	Bark, roots, leaves, fruit
71.	Arka	Calotropis gigantea (L.) br.	Under shrub	Root, latex, leaves, flowers
72.	Nimb!uka	Citrus medica L.	Small tree or shrub	Fruit, roo, bark
73.	Paṭola	Trichosanthes dioica Roxb	Climber	Fruits, leaves
74.	Aśoka	Saraca asoca (Roxb.) De wilde.	Tree	Bark

75.	Varuṇa	Crataeva nurvala Buch-Ham.	Tree	Bark, fruits, leaves
76.	Dhānya-Śāli	Coryza sativa Linn.	Tall herb (paddy crop)	Seed-grains
77.	Bakula	Mimusops elengi L.	Tree	Bark, fruits
78.	Āmra	Mangifera indica L.	Tree	Bark, fruits, flowers, leaves
79.	Jambu	Syaygium cumini (L.) Skeels	Tree	Fruit, bark, leaves
80.	Aśvattha	Ficus religiosa L.	Tree	Bark, leaves, fruits
81.	Vaṁśa	Dendrocalamus strictus Nees.	Tree	Leaves, shorts, roots, bark.
82.	Sanala-Śrīveṣṭaka	Pinus roxburghii Sarg.	Tree	Resin
83.	Kāśmarī	Gmelina arborea Roxb.	Tree	Bark, fruits
84.	Śyonāka	Croxylum indicum (L.) Vent	Tree	Root, bark, seeds.
86.	Kaṇṭakārī	Solanum surattense Burm. f. syn. Solanum xanthocarpum Schrad & Wendl.	Prostrate herb	Roots, whole plant
87.	Bṛhatī	Solanum indicum L.	Tall herb or under shrub	Roots, fruits

88.	Gokṣura	Tribullus terrestres L.	Prostrate herb	Fruit, whole plant
89.	Śalaparṇī	Desmodium gangeticum (L.) Dc.	Herb	Roots, whole plant
90.	Pṛśniparṇī	Uraria picta (Jacq.) Desv.	Herb	Roots, leaves, whole plant.
91.	Ativiṣā	Aconitum heterophyllum Wall	Herb	Rhizomes
92.	Tulasī	Ocimum sanctum L.	Herb	Leaves, roots, fruits
93.	Kṛṣṇa tulasī	Ocimum basilicum L.	Herb	Leaves, roots, fruits stems
94.	Vaṭa	Ficus bengalensis Linn.	Herb	Fruits stems
95.	Nirviṣī	Delphinium denudatumWall	Branched	Roots
96.	Pāṭhā	Cissampelos pareira Miers.	Climber	Roots, whole plant
97.	Surañjāna	Colchicum bluteum Baker	Herb	Bulb
98.	Vidārī	Pueraria tuberosa (Willd.) DC.	Twinning plant	Tubers
99.	Śatāvarī	Asparagus racemosus Willd.	Under shrub	Tuberous roots
100.	Āragvadha	Cassia fistula L.	Tree	Fruits, leaves, flowers, bark
101.	Pāribhadra	Erythrina indica Lamb	Tree	Flowers, fruits, bark
102.	Kākamācī	Solanum nigrum Linn.	Herb	Whole plant

103.	Rudravantī Rudanti	Capparis mooni Weight	Climber	Fruits
104.	Rasona	Allium sativum L.	Herb	Bulb, leaves
105.	Kāsamarda	Benincasa hispida (Thumb) cogn.	Twiner	Fruits
106.	Aparājita	Clitorea ternatea Linn.	Climber	Root
107.	Kanṭakikarañja	Caesalpinia crista Linn.	Shrub	Seeds
108.	Kumārī	Aloe vera L.	Succulent herb	Leaves
109.	Marica	Piper nigrum Linn.	Prostrate herb	Fruits
110.	Pippali	Piper longum L.	Prostrate herb	Fruits
111.	Gajapippalī	Scindapsus officinalis (Roxb.) Schott.	Climber	Fuits
112.	Pārasīka Yavānī	Hyoscyamus niger L.schott.	Herb	Seeds. leaves
113.	Agastya	Sesbania grandiflora Piers.	Tree	Flowers, roots
114.	Aśvagandha	Withania somnifera (L.) Dunal.	Under shrub	Roots

115.	Vṛddhadāru	Argyreia speciosa Sw.	Climber	Roots, leaves
116.	Apāmarga	Achyranthus aspera L.	Herb	Roots, whole plant, seeds
117.	Yavānī	Trachysperanum ammi (L.) Spr.	Herb	Seeds
118.	Suvarcala	Cleome gynandra L.	Under shrub	Roots, seeds, leaves
119.	Indravāruṇī	Citrullus colocynthis (L.) Schrad.	Twinner	Roots, fruits
120.	Vyāghrairaṇḍa	Jatropha curcas L.	Shrub	latex, stem
121.	Kaṭukā	Picrorrhiza kurroa benth.	Herb	Roots
122.	Madhuyaṣukā	Glycyrrhiza glabra Linn.	Herb	Roots
123.	Kākodumbara	Ficus hispida Linn.	Tree	Bark, fruits
124.	Dhattūra	Datura innoxia mill	Under shrub	Roots, seeds, leaves
125.	Drīpāntaravacā	Smilax glabra Roxb.	Climber	Roots, leaves
126.	Tvak	Cinnamomum zeylanicum Bl.	Tree	Bark, leaves
127.	Kupīlu	Strychnos nuxvomica L.	Tree	Fruit-seeds, roots, bark
128.	Vatsanābha	Aconitum ferox (Bruhl.) Muk	Herb	Roots
129.	Nārikela	Cocos nucifera L.	Truit	Fruits, roots

130.	Ḍāḍima	Punica granatum L.	Small tree	Fruits, root, leaves, stem
131.	Mūlaka	Raphanus sativus L.	Herb	Roots, pods, leaves
132.	Irīmeda	Acacia farnesiana (L.) Willd.	Tree	Bark, roots, pods
133.	Arjuma	Terminalia arjuna U&A.	Tree	Bark
134.	Devadāru	Cedrus deodara (Roxb.) Loud.	Tree	Wood-stem
135.	Mahānimba	Melia azedarach Linn..	Tree	Fruit-seeds, leaves, bark
137.	Palāá	Butea monosperma (Lamk.) Taub.	Latey	Plant
138.	Giriparpaṭa	Podophyllum hexandrum Royle	Herb	Rhizome
139.	Amila	Hippophae salicifolia Don.	Shrub	Bark
140.	Lalijarhi	Geranium nepalense Sw.	Herb	Root
141.	Sirīsqa	Albizzia lebbeck Benth	Tree	Bark, seeds
142.	Kuṣṭha	Saussurrea lappa C.B. Clarke.	Herb	Roots

143.	Tasvaya	Caragna cuneata	Herb	Whole plant
144.	Vārāhī	Dioscorea bulbifera Linn.	Climber	Bulb
145.	Madyantikā	Lawsonia inermis Linn.	Shrub	Leaves
146.	Balā	Sida cordifolia Linn.	Herb	Roots
147.	Dantī	Baliospermum montanum Muell.-Arg.	Shrub or herb	Roots, seeds
148.	Śallakī	Boswellia serrata Roxb.	Tree	Oleo-gum resin
149.	Saptaparṇa	Alstonia scholaris R. Br.	Tree	Bark
150.	Karavīra	Nerium indicum Mill.	Small tree or shrub	Bark
151.	Sītāphala	Anona squamosa Linn.	Small tree	Seeds, bark
152.	Jīvantī	Leptandenia reticulata W.&A.	Climber	Root. fruits
153.	Antammūla	Tylophora asthamatica W.&A.	Climber	Roots
154.	Caṅcu	Corchorus aestuans Linn.	Herb	Roots, whole plant
155.	Dugdhikā	Euphorbia hirta Linn.	Herb	Whole plant
156.	Sahadevī	Vernonia cinerea Linn.	Herb	Root

157.	Kālājāji	Nigella sativa Linn.	Herb	Seeds
158.	Pārijāta	Nyctanthes arbor-tristis Linn.	Small tree	Leaves, Bark
159.	Hastiśundī	Heliotropium indicum Linn	Herb	Whole plant, roots
160.	Miśreya	Forniculum vulgare Mill.	Herb	Seeds
161.	Sāla	Shorea robusta Gaertn.		Śalasāra (Olesigum resin)
162.	Priyāla	Buchonania lanzan Spreng	Tree	Seeds
163.	Bīyjaka	Pterocarpus marsupium Roxb.	Tree	Wood, resin
164.	Badara	Zizyphus mauritiana Lamk.	Small tree	Bark, fruit, leaves
165.	Gāṇgerukī	Grewia tenax Fiori	Shrub	Root, bark
166.	Dhanvayāsa	Fagonia cretica L.	Herb	Whole plant, leaves
167.	Dhātakī	Woodfordia fruiticosa Kurz.	Shrub	Flowers, bark
168.	Bākucī	Psoralea corylifolia Linn.	Herb	Seeds
169.	Kṛṣṇajīraka	Carum bulbocastanum W. Koech.	Herb	Fruits, seeds
170.	Kāśa	Saccharum spontaneum Linn.	Tall grass	Root

171.	Kāravī	Carum carvi Linn.	Herb	Whole plant
172.	Madhūka	Madhuca longifolia (Koen) Mac.	Tree	Bark, fruits
173.	Kuśa	Desmostachya bipinnata (Linn.) Stapf.	Herb-grass	Roots
174.	Mustaka	Cyperus rotundus Linn	Herb	Roots
175.	Viṣnukrāntā	Evolvulus alsinoides (L.) Linn.	Herb	Whole plant
176.	Sauvīra badara	Zizyphus sativa	Shrub	Fruits
177.	lavaṅga	Syzygium aromaticum (L.) Merr.	Shrub	Fl. buds
178.	Rāsnā	Pluchea lanceolata C.B. Clarke.	Herb	Roots
179.	Dūrvā	Cyndon dactylon (L.) Pers.	Grass	Whole plant
180.	Usaka	Dorema ammoniacum D.Don	Herb	Resinous gum
181.	Uśīra	Vetiveria zizanioides (L.) Nash	Grassy herb	Roots

182.	Cakramarda	Cassia tora Linn	Herb	Leaves, seeds, roots,
183.	Sūraṇa	Amorphophallus campanulatus Blume.	Blume	Herb Tuber campanulatus
184.	Nāgakeśara	Mesua ferrea Linn	Shrub	Seeds, flowers, woods,
185.	Keśara	Crocus sativus Linn	Herb	Fl-stigma
186.	Cavya	Piper chava Hunter	Climber	Fruits
187.	Ajamoda	Carum roxburghianum (DC.) Craib.	Herb	Seeds
188.	Māyāphala	Quercus infectoria Oliver	Tree	Galls
189.	Palakyā	Spinacea oleracea L.	Leafy herb	Plant, leaves, seeds
190.	Methikā	Trigonella foenum-graceum Linn	Herb	Seeds
191.	Dhānyaka	Coriandrum sativum Linn.	Herb	Fruit, leaves, plant
192.	Kampillaka	Mallotus philippinensis Muell-Arg.	Tree	Fruit-dust
193.	Gṛñjana	Daucus carota L.		Tuberous roots, seeds, leaves
194.	Jīraka	Cuminum cyminum Linn	Herb	Seeds

195.	Sarsapa	Brassica campestries Linn	Herb	Seeds, leaves
196.	Indrayava	Holarrhena antidysenterica Wall.	Tree	Seeds
197.	Vāstuka	Chenopodium allbum Linn	Herb	Whole plants, leaves
198.	Kāravellaka	Momordica charantia Linn	Climber	Fuits
199.	Taṇḍulīyaka	Amaranthus spinosus L.	Herb	Roots, leaves
200.	Patragobhi	Brassica capitata Linn. var oberacia .	Herb	cabbage
201.	Dhāmāṛgava	Luffa cylindirica (Linn.) M. J. Roem.	Clinber	Fuits
202.	Godhūma	Triticum aestivum L.	Tall herb (cereal)	Grains
203.	Raktavrntāka	Lycopersicon esculentum Mill syn. Lycopersicon lycopersicum (L.) Karst.	Herb	Fuits
204.	Āḍhakī	Cajanas cajan (Linn.) Millsp.	Under shrub	Seed-pulse, leaves
205.	Mudga	Vignaa radiata (Linn.) wilceek	Tall herb	Seeds
206.	Masura	Lens culinaris Medic	Tall herb	Seeds
207.	Caṇaka	Cicer arietinum Linn.	Herb	Leaves, seeds
208.	Śamī	Prosopis cineraria Druce	Tree	Bark, pods, leaves

209.	Ketakī	Pandanus fascicularis Lamk	Shrub	Roots, flowers, leaves
210.	Mucakunda	Pterospermum acerifolium Willd	Tree	Flowers, Bark
211.	Karpura	Cinnamomum camphora Nees	Tree	Bark, leaves,
212.	Vananimbuka	Glycosmis pentaphylla Correa	Shrub	Leaves
213.	Nagadamana	Pedilianthus tithimeloides Poir	Herb	Whole
214.	Lajjālu	Mimosa pudica Linn.	Prostrate herb	Seeds, roots
215.	Vanapsikā	Viola odorata L.	Herb	Whole plant
216.	Sthouneyaka	Taxus baccata Linn.	Tree	Leaves
217.	Ginseng	Panax ginseng C.A. Meyer Aralia pseudo-ginseng	Herb	Roots
218.	Jatāmāṁsī	Nardostachys jatamansi (Don) Dc.	Herb	Roots
219.	Rājikā	Brassica juncea (L.) czern.	Herb	Seeds, oil
220.	Alarka	Solanum trilobatum		
221.	Jātīphala	Myristica fragrans Houtt.	Small tree	Fruits

222.	Kośātaki -Tumbiû	Luffa acatangula (Linn.) Roxb.	Climber	Fruits
223.	Kārpāsa	Gossypium herbaceum L.	Shrub	Root, bark, seeds
224.	Soma	Ephedra gerardiana Wall	Herb	Root, stems
225.	Lankā	Capsicum annuum Linn.	Herb	Fruit, bark
226.	Sasmula-Hamuli	Elytraria acaulis (Linn.f.) Lindau.	Herb	Roots
227.	Vṛścikapatrī	Tragia involucrata L.	Shrub	Leaves, plant
228.	Vṛścikapatrī	Urtica dioica L.	Shruby herb	Leaves, roots
229.	Kokilākṣa	Hygrophilla auriculata syn. Astercantha longifolia Nees.	Herb	Seeds
230.	Nīlapuṣpī- (Fulanini)	Ageratum conyzoides Linn.	Herb	Leaves, flowers
231.	Dhava-Gabdi	Anogeissus latifolia Bedd.	Small tree	bark, other
232.	Iśvarī	Aristolochia indica L.	Climber	Plant
233.	Koinine	Brucea mollis Mall.ex Kunz (Simarubaceae)		Fruit, seeds
234.	Sabenbu kbenesing	Casearia vareca Roxb.		Fruits, leaves

236.	Gonga	Cochleospermum religiosum (L.) Alston	Tree	Bark, flowers, fruits, bark
237.	Anantamula	Hemidesmus indicus (L.) Br.	Climber	Roots
238.	Kṛṣṇa Sārivā	Ichnocarpus frutescens (L.) Br.	Cliber	Roots
239.		Dicranopteris linearis (Burm.f.) Underw syn. Gleichenia linearis Cl.		Fuits, roots
240.	Vanapalāṇḍu	Drimia indica (Roxb.) Fessop. syn. Uriginea indica (Roxb.) Kunth.	Herb	Bulb
241.	May¥uraśikhā	Elephantopus scaber L.	Herb	Root, plant
242.	Gilaphal	Entada purraetha Dc. syn. Entada phaseoloides (L.) Merr.		Plant
243.	Rusia-gach	Flemingia chappar Buch-Ham. ex Btn.		Seed, plant
244.	Hastikarna	Leea macrophylla Roxb.	Shrub	Roots, plant.

245.	Gogchapri	Eranthemum purpurascens Nees.	Herb	Roots, plant
246.	Sauvarcala-pīta	Cleome viscosa L.	Herb	Roots, leaves
247.	Śankhapuṣpī	Convolvulus pluricaulis Chois	Prostrate herb	Fruits,
248.	Saireyaka	Barleria prionitis Linn	Thorny herb	Leaves, flowrs, roots
249.	Kṛṣṇatulasī	Ocimum americanum Linn.	Herb	Various parts
250.	Māṁsarohiṅī	Somyda febrifuga A.Juss.	Tree	Bark
251.	Ikṣvāku	Lagenaria siceraria (Mol.) Standl.	Climber	Fruit

These herbal drugs are recommended, and used as medicine, food, diet, wholesome article, adjuvants and various other ways of utility considered as preventive and curative agent against cancer, based on system, texts, tradition, and medical practice supported with the studies and opened for interdisciplinary experiments, trials and investigatory researches in oncology.

SOME IMPORTANT ANTI-CANCER HERBAL DRUGS

1. Bhallātaka
2. Guggulu
3. Saptaparṇa
4. Brāhmī
5. Kāncanara
6. Devadāru
7. Vṛścikapatrī
8. Giriparpaṭa
9. Pāṣānabheda
10. Dāruharidrā
11. Caṅcu
12. Arka
13. Dhattūra
14. Maṅjiṣṭha
15. Pāribhadra
16. Sauvarcalā
17. Vanapsikā
18. Guḍūcī
19. Śirīṣa
20. Gunjā
21. Sitaphala
22. Śatāvarī
23. Sthouṇeyaka
24. Vaśā
25. Aśvagandhā
26. Āragvadha
27. Maṇḍūkapaṛṅī
28. Punarnavā
29. Bhṛṅgarāja
30. Pāṭhā
31. Bhumyāmalakī
32. Dhātakī
33. Aśvagandhā
34. Āmalakī
35. Kaṭukā
36. Drākṣā
37. Nirguṇḍī
38. Dāḍima
39. Śaṭī
40. Kuṣṭha
41. Palāśa
42. Haridrā
43. Babbula
44. Amaravallī
45. Āmragandhiharidrā
46. Araṇyaharidrā
47. Vacā
48. Akṣoṭa
49. Priyaṅgu
50. Parpaṭa
51. Saharramūla
52. Amisa
53. Śveta Rohitaka-(Rohitakajāti)
54. Vanya Nimbūka
55. Kapikacchu
56. Citraka
57. Harītakī

The relevant details of some important anticancer herbal drugs obtained from plant sources have been incorporated in forthcoming enumeration which has been presented in precise form and arranged in order of the names of plant species finding their utility as anticancer herbal agent belonging to the cadre of major potential drugs.

1. Abrus precatorius Linn

Papilionaceae (Fabaceae)

Guṅjā (Āyurveda)

Gunj, Ghungachi, Gomchi, Ratti (Hindi/common names)

Wild Liquorice Root, Crabes Eye (English)

Deciduous climber, with slender, flexible and tough branches. Leaves paripinate, rhachis byond the last pair of leaflets as a soft bristles; leaflets 10-20 pairs, opposite, linear-oblong, thingly membranous. Flowers, pink, clustered, usually leaf-bearing, axillary. Pods turgid, seed 3-6, ovoid, scarlet will a black spot at the hilium, polished bright, small-pea sized. Roots sweetish. Flowering and fruiting during autumn to winter season.

The plant is occurring wild throughout India upto 3,500 feet altitude. The seeds of plant contain abrin (N-Dnethyl-1-cryptophan). Two new alkaloids, the methyl ister of N,N-dinethyl-cryptophan-metho-cation and picatorin, in addition to abrin, hypaphorine and trigoneline reported from the seeds. Seeds coat contains a red colouring substance.

A protein extract obtained from the seeds exhibited anti-tumour activity against sarcoma (solid and ascites forms) in rats and fibrosarcoma in mica. Out of the various fractions of purified proteins of the seeds studied for antitumour activity in rats only the fraction (A5B) possessed anticancer activity.

The fruit has high content of vitamin C. Seeds contain fixed oil, essential oil and phasphates. Fruit, leaves and bark are rich in tanning. Fruits contain various other chemical constituents.

The fruits Emblica officinalis Gaertn. (hatrī) are used in medicine. they are also included among dietic items in various forms - The fruits (seedless pulp) form a major drug in indigenous systems of medicine. The drug is widely used in a number of diseases and it is a component of commonly used trio-group of myrobalans (triphatā) 1 or three Myrobalans). It is a restoralive (rasāyana) drug with preventive and curative properties. In general, the drug is useful in diseases of digestive system, reopiratory, urinary system, liver and nervous system. The drug is therapentically used in several other diseases in various forms and modes. It is employed in several formulations frequently prescribed in treatment of various ailments.

The drug is considered to possess anticancer activity. It is considered to be useful against cancer.

The seeds, roots and leaves of Gunjā (Abrus precatorius) are used in medicine. The seeds are toxic. Seeds are grouped in category of auxil!ary or secondary poisons (uparisṣa) in Indian medicine recommending its therapentic use for oral administration after due purification (śodhana).

The seeds are externally applied on chronic ulcer, alopecia, crysepalas leprosy, skin diseases and other similar eutaneous affections. the oil prepared with seeds is used in treating sinus, tumour, polypus, chronic wound, cervical ademitis, serophule, leprosy, scabics and other diseases. The leaves are used in different forms in rheumatic disorders, stomatitis and paralysis. The roots in sore throat and cough. The seeds are also useful as aphrodisiac and considered to be contraceptive (in female subjects).

The drug is considered to possess anticancer activity and it is useful in treatment of cancer.

2. Acacia nilotica ssp. indica (Benth.) Bremen.

syn. Acacia arabica willd.

Mimosaceae

Babbūla (Āyurveda)

Babul, Kikar, Bammr (Hindi/common names)

Small tree with bark of dark and brown colour or longitudinally fissured bark. Branchlets slender, terete, pubescent in young age. Leaves 2-pinnate, 5-10cm. long stipular spines very variable, 0.6-5cm. long, smooth, usually whitish, straight sharp, often absent; pinnae 4-9 pairs. Flowers yellow, in globose heads; peduncle axillary in fascicles of 2-8, terete, pubescent. Pods stalked, 7.5-15 by 1.5-1.6

cm., monoliform, compressed, constricted at the sutures between the seeds, densely and persistently grey downy, seeds 8-12. Flowering and fruiting during the period from summers to winters.

Plant is occurring throughout the greater part of India and various other countries in Asia and Africa. Common plant species for afforestation and a major forest component of dry and warmer (arid and xesophytic) zones of countιy.

The bark contains tannin and the leaves and fruits contain tannin 25%. Pods contain tannin 42%. Gum contains arabic acid, malic acid, sugar, enzyme and auxins.

The bark, gum, flowers and pods are used in medicine in various forms. The drug is potent astringent, and used in various diseases. Different parts of the drug plant area used in various forms and modes, as a single drug as well as in combination with other ingredient drugs. There medicinal recipes are administered both externally and internally. In general, the drug is useful in bowel, liver brain, urinary, veneral and respiratory complaints. It is used in uterine and vaginal discharges, skin diseases, fever, blood impurity and biliousness. Externally it is applied in wounds, burns, haemorhage, opthalmia, fracture and ulcerations. Vaginal douche is administered in vaginal and uterine complaints and the gargle is given in mouth and throat affections. Gum acacia is used for castor oil ermullsion given in dysentery and the gum is used in various other medicinal purposes.

The drug is considered to possess anticancer properties and it is useful in treatment of cancer.

3. Acorus calamus Linn

Araceae

Vacā (Āyurveda)

bach, Ghurhabach, barre, Vacha (Hindi/common names)

Calamus, Sweet Flag (English)

Erect, leafy perennial herbs, with thick and creeping root stock. Leaves large, tufted, ensiform, margins wavy. flowers minute. yellow-green, in 6-7 cm. long spaths. Perianth-segments 6, free. Stamens 6. Berries yellow-green, angular 1-3 seeded.

Plant is occurring throughout India and Sri Lanka ascending to 6000 feet altitude in tropical and substropical regions in the Himalayan retgions (upto 2000 meters). It grows in marshy and swampy places and along the rivers, rivulets and ponds or water-logged places. It is also planted and put under cultivation in certain areas with suitable habitat.

The rhizomes yield a volatile oil (1.5 to 3.5 percent) which contains chiefly asaryb aldehyde consisting two active principles (asarone). It also contains acorin, a bitter glucoside, eugemol, caffeine, starch and lesser quantity of tannin.

The rhizomes are used in medicine. The drug is useful as analgesic and anti-inflammatory, cariminative, stomachic, diuretic nervine tonic, diaphoretic and expectorant. It is intellect and memory promotor (medhya rasāyana) and hypotensive. The drug is used in various diseases and in health as psychosomatic protective medicine. It is an ingredient of some important compound formulations used in Indian medicine.

The drug is considered to possess anticancer properties and it is used in treatment of cancer.

4. Adhatoda zeylanica A. Medic

syn. Adhatoda vasica Nees., Justicia adhatoda L.

Acanthaceae

Vās˜(Āyurveda)

Vasa, Arhusa, Basing (Hindi/common names)

Evergreen shrubs, 1-2.5 meters high with feetid small, sometime taller. Leaves ovate, lanceolate, acute or acuminate at apex, narrowed at base. Flowers crowded in axillary spikes, towards the ends of branches. Corolla 2-2.5 cm. long, white with pink or purple streaks on the throat, bilabiate, filaments 2. capsules clavate, subacute, upto 2.5 cm. long. Seeds usually four. flowering and fruiting from December to May (or flowering in autumn season).

Plant is occurring commonly in hedges, wastelands, stonny land, scrub forests and roadside almost throughout India, ascending to 1,204-1,300 meters in the Himalayas generally in tropical and sub-tropical regions.

The leaves and root-bark contain wasicine, a crystalline alkaloid and very bitter substance. Leaves also yield adhatodic acid, a volatile oil and other chemical constituents.

The leaves, flowers, root-bark and whole plant (various parts) are useful in medicine. The drug is a valuable remedy for various ailments of respiratory system as an excellent expectorant, branchodilator and antispasmodic herbal agent. It is frequently given in treatment of cough, bronchitis, asthma and all chest diseases. the leaves and other parts of plant are employed as common igredient of cough syrups and other compuonds prescribed and marketed, specially indicated in chest and throat complaints. Similarly it is an ingredient in several classical formulations prepared and used in therapeusis of Indian medicine. The drug is used in pthisis (yakṣmā), intrinsic haemorrhage (raktapitta), fever, flatulence and other ailments.

The drug is considered to possess anticancer properties as it is recommended in chest cancer. Given specifically for checking the compliodious in stage of blood vomiting and other symptoms.

5. Allizzia lebbeck (linn.) Benth.

Caesalpiniaceae

Śirīṣa (Āyurveda)

Siras, Siris, sirash (Hindi/common name).

A large deciduous tree distributed upto 1200 meters in hilly region of Uttar Pradesh. it is one the common trees in India.

The tannins and psreudotannins, friedelin and r-ritosterol are found in the bark. The saponins based on echimocystic acid have been repoted.

The alcoholic extract of the roots has been found to possess anticancer activity in human epidermal carcinoma.

6. Alstonia scholaris (Linn.) R. Br.

Apocynaceae

Saptapaṇa (Ayurveda)

Tall or medium-sized evergreen tree, occurring between the elevation of 300-1000 meters in the Himalayan region of Uttar Pradesh.

Stem bark is highly medicinal. Bark contains a large number of alkaloids such as echitamine, echitenine, echitamidine, ditamine, scholarine, picrinine and non-nacrogenous substances amyurin and lupeol. The root is bitter tonic, alterative and febrifuge. The miley juice of plant is externally applied on ulcers. The alcoholic extract of the stam bark is found to possess anticancer activity in human sarcoma in the embryonated egg.

7. Anona squamosa Linn.

Annonaceae

Sitaphala

The plant contains a large number of compunds anonaine, reomerine, norcordine, cordine, norisocorydine, isocorydine, glaucine (+)-xylopine, (+)-o-mehydrmepavine, lanuginosine.

Amongst above aporine alkaloids anonaine, recmerine, norcordyne and corydine reported to ahve anticancer activity against human epidermal carcinoma of the naasopharynsxc in tissue culture.

8. Aphanamixis polystachya (Wall.) Parker

syn. Amoora rohitaka W.&A.

Meliaceae

Rohitaka jāti-bheda, Śveta Rohitaka (Āyurveda)

Awawatong, Harinhara, Tictaraj (Hindi/common names)

An evergreen tree, 30-60 ft. high; young parts finely silky. leaves large, imparipinnate, 1-2.5 ft. long; leaflets opposite, 4-8 pairs and an old one, 3-9 by 1-1/3-4 in., elliptic-oblong or oblong-lanceolate, acuminate, glabrous on both surfaces, very inequilateral, obtuse or acute at the base; petiolules 1/4-1/3 in long.

Male flowers numerous erect 1/6 in. long, subglobular, in solitary, axillary panicles more than half as long as the leaves. Female or Hermasohrodite flowers larger than the males, in axillary or supra-axillary solitary spikes much shorter than the leaves.

Fruit 1-1.5 in in diam., globular, yellow when ripe; pericarp coriaceous, smooth, 3-celled, opening by 3 valves. Seeds oblong with a scarlet aril. Flowering in July.

Plant is occurring in India, western peninsula, Assam, Oudh and other regions. the bark of plant drug is mainly 8used in medicine and some other parts like seeds and leaves are also medicinally useful. Bark is used in live complaints, pain after child birth or post-nateal pain (makkalaś¥ula), spleen disorders, teeth problems and some other diseases. Seeds are used in rheumatic complaints. Leaves are fish poison and bark gives a green dye.

The drug is reported to possess anticancer activity and it is recommended to be useful in treatment of cancer.

The plant Amoora rohituka W&A has been studied and the drug belongs among various drugs available in ancient literature of medical science which drawn attention of scientists working on various aspects of anticancer herbal agents and several drugs and their preparations have been investigated.

The observations and results indicated that the bark of Amoora rohitaka was found particulary to be effective against cancer.

The results of earlier investigations revealed its anti-leucocytic and anti-lymphocytic activity, immunosuppressive activity and anticancer activity by cell electrophorotic studies has resulted in the solution of the active principle showing significant anti-tumor ac6tivity on expermental mommary tumor in vitro.

Anti-tumor studies on a new herbo-mineral have been conducted recently (Prasad, G.C. et pal, JRAS, vol. XX, No. 1-2, 1999, pp. 10-19). Based on the anti-tumor activity of the ethanolic extract of the bark of Amoora rohitaka W.&A., the bio-active component was isolated to be prieurianin, a limonoid of this plant. A new complex of copper 9II) acetate and prieurianin [cu (prieu) (acetate) has been tested against L-929 fibroblast (murine tumor cell), P-815 (murine mastocytoma, Raji - Burkitt-Lympho (human tumor cell) and wahi Abelson virus (human induc ed monocytic cell). Prieurianin also showed significant cytotoxic activity against experimental mammary tumors.

The chemical characterisation of the active principle of the plant drug has importance in view of anti-cancer activity of chemical constituents which are found active biologically and pharmacologically in conditions of cancerous problems.

The drug plant Amoora rohitaka W.&A. has been found a rich source of limonoids and several prieurianin-type limonoids other than prieurianum itself have been isolated from the seeds of this plant. The stem barkof Amoora rohitaka has also been investigated, but the limnoids reported from the bark are considered relatively simple.

The isolated active principle PM 209-11°C should in its FBA mass specturm a sodium adduction at m/g 785 which corresponds to the molecular weight 762 and led to the determinatin of its molecular formula as $C_{38} H_{50} O_{16}$ on the basis of the results of elemental analysis.

The spectral features of the compound revealed it to be a close relative of Rohituka rorale, a constituent of the seeds of the plant. Various spectral data are studied disclosing the presence of investigation for characteristic functionlities of active principle as an anti-tumor agent which has the area of prospects after further study as anticancer drug on clinical level in human subjects.

9. Asparagus racemosus Willd.

Liliaceae

Śatāvarī (Āyurveda)

Shatavar, Shataur, Shatavari (Hindi/common names)

A climbing shrub, distributed all over the region of Uttar Pradesh hills between the elevation of 1500-2100 meters.

The alcoholic extract of the roots have been found to possess anti-cancer activity in human epidermal carcinoma of the nasopharynx in tissue culture.

The roots contain saponins which on hydrolysis yields sarsopogenin, glucose and rhamnose.

The roots are highly mucilaginous, refrigerant, nutritive tonic, demulcent and galactogogue. Locally the roots are used in healing ulcers. It is a valuable drug used in medicine.

Other species of Asparagus possessing medicinal properties are worthmentioning: Asparagus curillus Asparagus fillicinus, Asparagus gracilis and Asparagus adscendens.

10. Bacopa monnieri (L.) Pennel.

Scrophulariaceae

Brāhmi, Aindrī

Brahmi, Birmi, Jalnim, Brahmi Booti

Prostrate, succulent herbs; annual, sem-aquatic, branches spreading or ascending and rooting at the nodes. Leaves obovate-oblong or apathulate upto 18mm. long. Flowers companulate bluish-purple or white with bluish veins, solitary, oxillary, short or long, pedicellate. Capsules glabrous, ovoid, tipped with persistent style. Flowering and fruiting in August-September.

Plant is distributed in the Himalayan region upto an elevation of 1200 meters.

The alkaloids brahmine, herpestine are repoted in earlier phytochemical investigations. Besides these alkaloids betulic acid, sigmasterol, B-sitosterol, d-memitol and two types of sapnins namely Bacoside A and Bacoside B are found in further screenings which record other data on chemical constituents.

The aleoholic extract of the whole plant possesses anticancer activity in human epidermal carcinoma of the nasopharynx in tissue culture.

Whole plant is used in medicine. It is generally collected during winter season. Plant is a prominent and valuable herbal drug possessing chief properties of nervine tonic, diuretic and blood purifier and its has presently become a memory enhancing (promoting) drug.

The crude material of brahmi in the form of dried whole plant is marketed and in raw drug trade.

11. Bauhinia varietaga L.

Bauhinia racemosa Lamk.

Caesalpiniaceae

Kāṅcanāra

Kochnar, Karale, Kaudi (Hindi and common names)

Small crooked deciduous tree distributed in sub-Himalayan tract of the region upto 1500 meters.

Small or medium-sized, deciduous trees. Leaves simple, sub-orbicular cordate, 11-15 nerved, divided to about 1/4 in way down. flowers white, with upper petal purplish, in axillary and terminal, few-flowered corymbose racemes. Pods flat, 10-25x1.5-2.5cm. glabrous. Flowering in February-April and fruiting in July-September.

The stem-bark is used in medicine. Flowering buds are consumed as vegetable after cooking. the bark is useful therapeutically in treatment of tumour, goitre, epistaxis, uterine bleeding and skin diseases.

Stem bark yielded stigma sterol, lupeol, naringenin and B-sitosterol. The alcoholic extract of the stem bark has been found to ahve anticancer activity against human epidermal carcinoma of the nasopharynse in tissue culture.

The raw material of Kachnar chal which is stem bark procured from trees of Bauhinia species is marketed under drug trade.

12. Berberis lycium Royle

Berberidaecae

Dāruharidrā (Āyurveda)

Large, spiny shrubs, upto 4 meters high. Stems pale, glabrous or pubescent. Spines 3-feet at base. Leaves oblanc3eolate to obovate, entire or 2-4 spinulate, greyish or whitish below. Flowers yellow, 7-8 mm. across, on elongate racemes. Berries ellipsoid to avoid, blue or black, covered with bloom, minutely stylose. Flowering in March-April and fruiting in May-July.

Plant is distributed in sub-tropical and temperate regions, between 800-2500 meters. Common throughout the Himalayan regions.

Roots, root-bark, stem and dried aqueous extract are mainly used in medicine. Fruits and flowers are also medicinal.

The drug is alterative, antimalarial, antiseptic, blood-purifier, and sedative. it is used in liver and spleen enlargement and other disorders, it is useful in anaemia and jaundice. The drug is useful in conjunctivitis, neuralgia, haemorrhoids, urogenital disorders, ulcers and other various diseases.

The alkaloid berberine and its salts obtained from roots are used in medicine. Berberine hydrochloride and sulphate are used in preparation of various drugs useful in cholera, diarrhoea, dysentery, eye troubles and oriental sores.

The roots and stem are water extracted for preparing Rasāṇjana (rasaunt) which is also marketed alongwith other parts medicinally useful.

Some other useful species of Berberis :

***Berberis asiatica* Roxb. ex DC.**

Berberidaceae

The roots contain berberine, berbamine, palmitine, farorshizine, columbamine, tetrahydropalmitine, oxyberberine and oxyacanthine. The root bark is tonic and antiperiodic while stem bark is diaphoretic and laxative.

Berberis aristata Dc.

Berberidaceae

The main important alkaloid is berberine. The root-bark is purgative, however, the plant is used as tonic, stomachic, astringent, anti-periodic, diaphoretic and alterative.

The main important alkaloid is berberine. The root-bark is purgative, however, the plant is used as tonic, stomachic, astringent, anti-periodic, diaphoretic and alterative.

***Berberis lycium* Royle.**

Berberidaceae

The roots contain umbellatine. This species is considered is rich source of berberine. The root is a febrifuge, carminative and gentle aperient.

The species of Berberis are reported to possess anti-cancer activity in human epidermal carcinoma of the nasopharynx in tissue culture.

Some other species of Berberis occurring in the Himalayan region are worthmentioning: Berberis chitria, Berberis floribunda, Berberis verlgaris, Berberis petiolaris and Berberis jacschkeana.

13. Bergenia ligulata (Wall.) Engl.

Saxifragaceae

Pāṣāṅabheda (Āyurveda)

A large thick-stemmed lithophytic herb common in moist rockty slopes or shady ravines of rocks distributed in temperate zones of area upto 2700 meters elevation. Temperate regions between 1800-3000 meters.

Perennial herbs. Rootstock thick, creeping. leaves large, thick, orbicular or obovate, margins fringed with short stiff hairs, stalk stem sheathing at the base. Flowers white, pink or purple, in spreading cymose panicles, terminating a flexible scape; calyse glabrous; petals 5; stamens 10 capsule 2-beaked. flowering in March-April. Rhizones collected in winter season. Bergenia ciliata (Haw.) Sternb. forma ligulata yeo. syn. Bergenia ligulata (Wall.) Engl., Sascifraga ligulata wall.

The chemical constituents bergenin and B-sitosterol have been reported. Other compounds from the roots isolated are gallic acid, tannic acid, glucose, mucilage and the wax.

The alcoholic extract of the roots possesses anticancer activity against walker carcinosacroma 256 in rats.

Rhizomes are used widely in medicine, specifically recommended in urinary diseases, urinary claculus, kidney stones, urinary bladder stones, dysuria, painful micturition and other similar urinary ailments (including prameh) and diabetes), heart diseases, piles and various other diseases. The paste of rhizome (fresh) is quite effective when applied on swellings, ulcer and abscess as the drug is wound-healter.

Other species of Bergenia occur in the Himalayan regions and medicinally useful are: Bergenia ciliata Royle and Bergenia stracheyi (Hook.f.& Thoms.) Engler.

14. Boerhavia diffusa L.

Nyctaginaceae

Punarnavā (Āyurveda)

Punarnava, Santhi (Hindi/common names)

Figweed (English)

Diffuse herbs with prostrate or ascending branches. Tap root stout. Leaves in unequal pairs, ovate or suborbicular, margins undulate. Flowers pink, minute, in small bracteate umbels of 4-10, arranged in long-stalked, axillary and terminal panicles. Perianth 10-lobed.

Fruits clavate, 5-toothed, viscidly, glandular on the roots. Flowering and fruiting in major part of the year.

Plant is occurring as weed throughout India. It grows wild in subtropical regions below 100 meters, frequently met with in wastelands, roodsides, open lands and grounds.

Plant contains punarnavine, a slightly bitter alkaloid (0.04 percent), potassium nitrate (0.52 percent) and other chemical constituents.

The roots, seeds, leaves and whole plant are used in medicine, especially roots. The drug is potent diuretic and important medicine used in disorders of urinary system. it is useful in oedema, liver disorders, heart diseases, anaemia, jaundice, cough, asthma, chest-wound, abdominal diseases, fever, debility and eye complaints.

The drug is considered to possess anticancer activity.

15. Butea monosperma (Lamk.) Kuntze.

Palāśa (Āyurveda)

Dhak, Taisu, Palas (Hindi/common names)

Flame of the forest (English)

Small or moderate-sized, deciduous trees, 6-8 meters high-leaves 3-foliolate; leaflets broadly, obovate or rhomboid. Flowers large, orange-red in fascicles on axillary and terminal racemes. Calyse dark-brown, velvety. Pods 10-20cm long, flat silky-tomentose. Flowering and fruting in March-July.

Plant is occurring throughout India specially warm regions and it is found in the subtropical regions in hilly areas upto 1000 meters.

The bark and gum contain kine-tannic acid and gllic acid 50%, mucilaginous substance and alkalies 2% Seeds contain an active principle, palasonin and seeds also yield fixed oil 18 percent.

The bark, flowers, leaves, gum (Butea-gum or Bengal-Kim) and seeds are used in medicine. Seeds are used as potent anthelmintic and given in round worm affections. Flowers are used as diruetic and aphrodisiac. The gum is useful as astringent and given in diarrhoea and dysentery. The flowers and seeds are useful in ringworm and skin diseases. The leaves are applied over inflammed and painful organs. Bark decoction is externally applied as formentation in ulcer, piles and vaginal discharge. Various parts of plant drug are useful in fracture, sexual impotency, general debility, poisons, dysuria, eye diseases, blood impurities, blood diseases, gout, leucorrhoea, fever, burning sensation scorpion string and epilepsy. Seeds are also useful as contraceptive.

The drug is considered to be useful in treatment of cancer.

16. Callicarpa macrophylla Vahl.

Verbenaceae

Priyaṅgu, Puṣpa Priyaṅgu (Āyurveda)

Phool priyangu, Priyangu, Dahiya (Hindi/common names)

Erect, evergreen shrub, 2-2.5 meters high-Branches, leaf-stalks and inflorescence densely wooly tomentose. Leaves opposite, shortly stalked, lanceolate, acuminate, crenate or sharply toothed, upper surface wrinkled, pubescent; lower tomentose. Flowers pink, hardly 5mm. long, crowded in axillary, dichotomous cymes. Fruits white, succulent, globose, containing 4 one-seeded nutlets. Flowering and fruiting during rainy season and winter season.

Plant is occurring in subtropical regions in wastelands and ravines upto 1200 meters. it is growing fairly common around hilly towns and other localities in lower hills and terai region.

The roots contain aromatic essential oil. Fruits and other parts contain various chemical substances.

The flowering buds or flowers are used in medicine. The drug is useful as haemostatic, blood purifier, astringent, cooling, better tonic, carminative, analgesic and antipyretic, it pacifies burning sensation and checks foul smell of body as well as over-sweatening. Externally it is applied to foul ulcers (bed smelling), chronic ulcers and skin affections. Leaves are used for fomentation in rheumatic organs. it is specially given in ailments caused by blood impurities.

The drug is consdiered to possess anticancer activity and it is used in treatment of cancer.

17. Calotropis gigantea R.Br.

Asclepiadaceae

Arka (Āyurveda)

Aka, Akha, Akaua (Hindi /common)

An erect shrub usually 1.8-2.4 meters high; young parts clothed with white cottony tomentum; bark soft, corky, spongy leaves subsessile, usually 5.7-1.5 by 4.5-8-2 cm. broadly ovate, ovate-oblong, elliptie, obovate, cottony, pubescent. Flowers in umbellate cymes, peduncled, buds globose. Follicles 7.5-10x5-7.5 cm., subglobose, ellipsed or avoid. Seeds 6 by 4mm, broadly ovate, acute.

Plant species are distributed upto 1200 meters elevation in Himalayan region. it is generally growing in waste lands and also in damp places. Plant is common throughout India in warm and dry places.

The leaves of plant Calotropis gigantea R. Br. contain the active principle mudarine. Besides this three glycosides present are colotropin, calotoxin and uscharin. The milky juice is a violent purgative.

Tthe alcoholic extract of leaves and roots ahve been found to possess anticancer activity against human epidermal carcinoma of the naso-pyharynx in tissue culture.

The plant calotropis procera R.Br. conains calotrophin. A powerful bacteriolytic agent (asclepin) is found to be present in the latex of this species. the milky juice of plant is applied topically for washing ulcers and wounds. The alcoholic extract of the roots and the leaves have been found to possess anticancer activity against human epidernal carcinoma of the nasopharynx in tessue culture.

18. Cassia fistula Linn

Āragvadha (Āyurveda)

Amaltas (Hindi/common names)

Indian Laburnum (English)

Small or medium-sized trees, 6-9 meters high, trunk straight; bark smooth and pale grey, rough. Leaves pinnately compound with leaflets 4-8 pairs, ovate to ovate-lanceolate or ovate-oblong, margins, entire, bright green and glabrous above, paler and silvery-pubescent beneath (when young). Flowers in lax racemes, bright or golden yellow, beautiful. Fruits cylindrio pods, 30-60cm. long, 2-2.5cm. diam., pendulous, nearly straight, green and turns dark brown-black (at ripening stage). Seeds embeded in pulp, compressed, completely reported, coins-shaped, many. Flowering and fruiting during to March to April and colder months.

The plant is occurring throughout India and other adjascent regions in Asian continents. it grows in tropical and subtropical regions in the Himalayan region ascending to 1200-1500 meters elevation. it is also an ornamental tree planted frequently in various regions of country.

The leaves contain anthraquinone derivatives. Root-bark contains phenes and oxyanthraquinone substance. pulp contains resinous and waxy and oily substance besides other various constituents.

Various parts of the plant are used in medicine: leaves, roots, bark, fruit-pods, fruit-pulp, root-bark and flowers.

The drug is useful in constepation, skin diseases, bowed and abdominal troubles, fever, cardiac and usinary disorders, biliousness, glandular diseases, goitre, rheumatic complaints, inflammation, blood impurities and skin diseases. Different parts are also used in treatment of various other diseases. They are employed in various formulations.

The drug is considered to possess anti-cancer effect and it is suggested to be used in various cancer conditions.

19. Cedrus deodara (Royle ex. D. Don.) G. Don.

Pinaceae

Devadāru(Āyurveda)

Large evergreen trees; branches and branchlets horizontal, tips slender and nodding. Leaves 2.5-3.8 cm. long, needle-shaped, 3-sided, glaucous green. Male and female flowers often on separate trees, but sometimes on the same trees, in which case they are on separate branches. Cones erect, barrel-shaped, 7.6-12.6 cm. long, 5-8.8cm. in diam.; scales numerous, fan shaped, imbricate. Seeds triangular. Flowering (male flowers) in September-October. cones ripening in October-November (after about one year of apperance).

It is distributed in the Himalayas between 1200 and 3600 meters. Very common in temperate zone of Himalayan region between 1800-300m. component of forest composition in various zones in the Himalaya.

The wood, bark and oil are medicinally useful. The bark is astringent and febrifuge. The alcoholic extract of the stem bark possesses inticancer activity against human epidermal carcinoma of the nasopharynx in tissue culture.

The wood yields on stem distillation a raddish-brown oil which is used as a substitute for cedar wood oil of commerce. The bark is considered as a good remedy in remittent and intermittent fevers, diarrhoea and dysentery. It is especially useful in bilious fevers and certain kind of diarrhoea. The oil obtained from wood is useful in ulcers, skin diseases and rheumatism.

The essential oil from the plant contains p-methylace cophenones p-methyl-tetrahydro-acetophenone and adantone; it also contains two sesquiterpenes namely a - and b- himachaline which constitute the major portion of the oil. A new sesquiterpenes himachalol related to himacholenes has also been reported in the oil.

20. Centella asiatica (L.) Urban. syn. Hydrocotyle asiatica L.

Apiaceac (Umbelliferae)

Maṇḍukparṇī (Āyurveda)

Brahmi, Mandukaparni (Hindi/common names)

Indian Pennywort (English)

Prostrate or creeping herbs, rooting at the nodes; annual or perennials. Leaves many at lach nodes, kidney-shaped, margins toothed. Flowers small, pink, in clusters of umbels, each cluster bearing 3 or 4 flowers. Fruits minute, laterally compressed. Flowering and fruiting during the period from April to October.

Plant fund in most places along water tanks, ponds, water river-beds, stream, ditches or semi-aquatic localities, almost throughout India, ascending to regions, upto 2000 feet and also upto 1500 meters in the sub-tropical Himalayan regions.

Herb contains alkaloid hydrocotyline. Fresh leaves yield asiaticoside -0.7-0.12 grains, a glycoside. Vallerine, yancunoside, asiatic acid, resin brahmicide and other several chemical constituents.

Whole herb and leaves are used in medicine. The drug is brain tonic, it is medhya-rasāyana (intellect-promoting and restorative) drug belonging to rejuvenating group (rasāyana) of drugs. It is useful in various psychosomatic diseases, skin complaints, leprosy, anaemia, jaundice, nervous disorders, mental disorders, debility and used as a hair tonic. It is useful is glandular leprosy, chronic ulcers, tubercular wounds, adenitis and other similar complaints.

The plant is considered to possess anti-cancer activity.

21. Cissampelos pareira L.

syn. Cissampelos pareira L. var. hirsuta

(Buch-Ham. ex. DC.) Forman.

Menispermaceae

Pāṭhā (Āyurveda)

Patha, Podhal, Kalipath, Padh (Hindi/common names)

Icevine, Pareira Brava (English)

Twinning shrubs, with grey-tomentose on glabrous branchlets. Leaves orbicular or broadly ovate, truncate or sub cordate at base, rounded at apex. Flowers small, greenish-yellow Male flowers in 5-6 cm. long, corymbose cymes. Female flowers clustered in the axils of orbicular bracts, forming pendulous racemes. Drups 2-4 mm. across, comprossed, scarlet when ripe. Flowering and fruiting in May-November.

The roots of plant contain pelosine or berberine (.5 percent) and also raponin. Other species yield other alkaloids.

The roots and aerial parts are used in medicine. The roots and leaves are used in chronic or foul ulcers, sinus, scabies, prurities, leprosy and other cutaneous affections. It is useful in dysentery, diarrhoea, dropsy, cough, urinary complaints and febrile conditions. The drug is useful to purify latex of mothers and as bitter tonic.

The drug plant is considered to be useful in cancer.

22. Cleome gynandra Linn.

Capparidaceae

Sauvarcala (Āyurveda)

Jakhiya, Talparni (Hindi/common names)

The seeds have anthelmintic properties. The alcoholic extract of the entire plant is found to possess anticancer activity against human epidermal carcinoma of the nasopharynx in tissue culture and hepatoma (129) in mouse.

A strong smalling weed is found abundantly in warmer/parts of the foot hills (Uttar Pradesh) and other regions.

23. Commiphora mukul (Hook.ex Stocks) Engl.

Bursearaceae

Guggulu (Āyurveda)

Gugal, Guggal (Hindi/common names)

Shrubs 1.2-1.3 meters high; young parts glndular-pubescent; branches knotty and crooked, divaricate usually ending in a sharp spin. Leaves 1-3-foliolate, leaflets subsessile, rhomboid-ovate, serrate-toothed in the upper part, smooty, shinning. Flowers in fascicles of 2-5, triangular, as long as the tube. Drupes 6-8 mm. diam., ovoid, acute; epicarp 4-valved; pyrenes ovate, readily splitting into two. Flowering and fruiting after rains and extending to autumn season.

Plant is occurring in warmer regions and deserts (also arid zones) of country, it grows wild in Rajasthan (Rajputana), Gujarat (Kathiawarh), Mysore, Deccan and other areas in India including ravines in Central India (M.P.-U.P. border).

The oleo-gum-resin which is an exudate of stem and trunk (when injured or incised) and used as drug after proper purification (śodhana) in medicine. It is of five kinds and some other varieties.

It contains a volatile oil, resinous gum a bitter active principle.

It is a major drug of Indian medicine. It is quite useful in vātavyādhi. The drug is used in rheumatic diseases, arthritis, cough, asthma, worms, opthalmia, obesity, tumour, cyst, heart troubles, dyspepsia, epilepsy, amenorrhoea, ocdema, goeitre, gout, sinus, ulcer, fistula and skin diseases. It is a rasāyana (restorative) drug. It is an ingredient of several formulations.

The drug is considered to possess anticancer activity; it is therapeutically recommended in management of arbuda (tumour) and various kinds of cancer in different forms and employed as component in various compounds used in treatment of cancer.

Thus, the drug is widely used for treatment of cancer and generally it is found to be major component of vrious compound formulation which are frequently prescribed for treating cancer and other diseases in indigenous system of medicine. Some classical formualtions (śāstrīya yoga) are noteworthy as follow :

A. 1. Kāncanāra guggulu
   2. Paṅcatikta guggulu
   3. Vraṇāri guggulu
   4. Kaiśoura guggulu
   5. Triphalā guggulu
   6. Pancavimiśati guggulu
   7. Yogarāja guggulu
   8. Other guggulu yogāh (compounds)

B. 1. Ārogyavardhini Vaṭī
   2. Candraprabhāvaṭī
   3. Other formulations containing guggulu

24. Corchorus aestuans Linn.

Tiliaceare

Cancu (Ayurveda)

Chinch, Chunch (Hindi/common names)

A common wead, annual herb in hotter parts of the country, particulary in sandy and grassy localities of river beds, field and roadises.

Erect or sub-erect, simple or slightly branched, pilose-hairy, annual herbs, upto 60 cm. tall. leaves ovate-lanceolate, to oblong, acute-sub acuminate at apex, rounded or subcordate at base, double serrate, pilose. Flowers pale-yellow, 1-3 together on short, axillary peduncles. Capsules 2-4cm. long, with 6,8 or 10 serrate, broad-winged angles. Seeds small, many. Flowering and fruiting in autumn season and onwards.

Numerous cardiac glycosides are found in the plant. These include monoxide and polar glycosides. The monoxide is characterised as helveticoside and corchoroside A. The two polar glycosides are erysimo-side and olicoside.

The alcoholic extract of the entire plant has been found to possess anticancer activity against epidermal carcinoma of the nasopharynsx in tissue culture.

Whole plant is demulcent. The leaves, fruits, seeds and entire herb are useful in medicine. Seeds and leaves are stomachic and mainly used in medicine. paste is externally applied to ulcers. Seeds are considered antiseptic. Leaves are useful as demulcent and useful in obdominal disorders. The fruits (seeds) are applied in the form of paste to sinus, chronic ulcers and other wounds.

Other species of Corchorus are also worth mentioning : Corchorus capsularis LInn., Corchorus oliotorus Linn. and Carehorus trilocularis Linn.

The drug is considered to be useful in treatment of cancer.

25. Curcuma amada Roxb.

Scitaminacear

Āmragandhiharidrā (Āyurveda)

Amahaldi, Saphedahaldi, Ambahaldi (Hindi/common names)

Mango-giner (English)

Annual herb, 60-100cm., resembling turmeric plant. Rootstock large, sessile, tubers thick, cylindric or ellipsoid, pale-yellow inside. Leaves long petiolate, in tufts, blade oblong-lanceolate, acute or acuminate, glabrous and green on both, sides. Flowers in autumnal spikes, flowering bracts greenish white, tinged with pink or red. Rootstock smelling like mango fruit and appearing (in shape) like ginger; rhizomes sympodial. Flowering and fruiting during autumn season.

Plant is occurring in West Bengal, Orissa, Southern and Western India and Western Peninsula.

The rhizomes yield an aromatic essential il which contain several chemical substances like curcumin, myristic acid and some other components responsible for mango-odour.

The rhizomes are useful as stomachic, appetizer, anodyne mervine tonic, astringent, anti-prutitic, and antiphlogistic and laxative. The ghizomes are known remedy against sprains, contrusions, trauma and other painful as well as swollen lesions. It is also applied to skin diseases, itch, scabies, ulcers, srores and other cutaneous affections.

The drug is considered to possess anticancer properties and it is useful in treatment of cancer. The drug is reported to have anti-tumour action and utility.

26. Curcuma aromatica Salish.

Scitaminaceae

Araṇyaharidrā, Vanyaharidra (Āyurveda)

Benhaldi, Kepurhaldi, Janglihaldi (Hindi/common names)

Herb looking like tumeric plant, with large rootstock, palmately branched sessile, annulate biennial tubers, yellow and aromatic inside, polats-like rhizomes with camphorous odour. Leaves oblong-elliptic or oblong-lancolate, green, often variegated above, pubescent beneath, petioles as long as or longer than the blade. Flowering sem appearing with or before the leading stem. Flowers fragrant, shorter than the bracts, in spikes, pale green, funnel shape, lip yellow. Flowering and fruting during summer season and onwards.

Plant is occurring almost throughout India particularly in Mysore and Malabar forests. It is cultivated in various parts of country specially West Bengal, Souther India, Karnataka and other regions.

The rhizomes contain volatile oil, resin, white substance, mucilaginous matter, sugar exudation, yellow colouring matter, albuminoides and an active substance cucumin. Aromatic oil of rhizomes yield various odorous substances.

The rhizomes (root stock) are used in medicine. The drug is useful as anti-inflammatory, analgesic, anti-tumor, blood purifier antidermatitis carminative, tonic, stomachic and antidote to venomous poison. Externally the rhizomes are applied on skin diseases, erruptions, scabies, leucoderma, bruises, tumours, sprains, trauma, inflammed and painful lesions (organs) and snake-bite (also given internally). it has antifungal and antispasmodic properties. it has also utility as spice.

The drug is considered to possess anticancer activity, it has antitumour action. It is useful in treatment of cancer.

27. Curcuma longa Linn

Scitaminaceae

Haridrā (Āyurvedā)

Haldi, Haladi, Hardi, Haradi (Hindi/common names)

Turmeric (English)

Tall herb with large and ovoid root stock attaching sessile cylindric tubers, orange-coloured inside. Leaves very large, in tufts (upto 1.2 meters long or more) including the petiole as long as the blade). Flowers in autumnal spikes, 10-15cm. long, peduncle 15cm. long or more, concealed by the sheathing petiole, flowering bracts pale-green, bracts of coma tinged with pink. Flowering in autumn or farming season.

Plant is cultivated throughout tropical regions and in other regions including hilly areas. It is under commercial farming for production and trade of spice.

The rhizome contains a volatile oil, an active principle curcumin, yellow colouring matter and turmeric oil (turmeriol).

The rhizomes are used in medicine. Rhizome has major use as a common spice. As a drug the rhizomes in fresh as well as dried form are used in medicinal recipes as a single drug as well as they are employed in compound formulations. the drug is used in skin, blood (impurity), pigmentation, worms, respiratory and allergic disorders. It is effective as an astringent, haemostatic, wound healer analgesic and antiseptic drug. It is useful in liver disorders, jaundice, urinary and catarrhal affections. Externally, the drug is used in wounds, injuries, dental and gums troubles, sprains and blood haemorshage (cuts and injuries).

The drug is considered to possess anti-cancer activity and it is used in treatment of cancer.

28. Cuscuta reflexa Roxb.

Convolvulaceae / Cuscutaceae

Amarvallī Ākāśavallī (Āyurveda)

Amarbel, Akashbel (Hindi/common names)

Dodder (English)

Leafless twining parasitic plant. Stems brown or yellow, branches fleshy stout, forming dense, yellow masses on the host covering by its net of thread-like stems and branches. Flowers sessile or very shortly pedicalled, in clusters, arranged in racames, fleshy, solitary or in clusters, often warty. Capsules globose; seeds 2-4 black, large in small fruits.

Plant is occurring throughout India and it is commonly found on host-hedges, shrubs herbs and small trees.

Plant contain quercetion, resin cuscutin and amrvelline and other chemical substances.

The whole plant and seeds are used in medicine. The drug is astringent, alterative, anthelmintic, purgative and cardiac tonic. it is useful in dyspepria, flatulence, liver and bilary disorders, fever and urinary complaints; it is also useful in pthisis, gonorrhoea, seminal disorders, painful micturition, general debility, worms and protracted fevers. Externally an infusion of whole herb is applied as wash-lotion for rores, itch and scabies. The juice of plant is used as an eye-drop in conjuctivitis. Plant is applied on acute pain of organs and it is also used in hair diseases. Juice is applied to ulcers and inflammed parts of body. The herb is blood purifier, antirheumatic, diuretic and wound healer.

Another plant Cassytha filiformis Linn. (belonging to family Lauraceae) is known as Ākāśavalli or Amaravallī. Some other species of genus Cuscuta (belonging to family Cuscutaceae) are medicinally useful : Cuscuta capitata Roxb., C. Chinensis Lam. and C. hyalina Roth.

The drug is considered to possess anticancer acvitity and the herb is used in treatment of cancer. It has also been reported that Cuscuta chinensis Lam. (whole plant) is useful in treating cancer.

29. Datura stranonium L.

Solanaceae

Dhatt¥ura (Āyurveda)

Dhatura (Common/Hindi)

Thorn Apple (English)

Bushy erect annuals, upto 1 meters tall. Leaves large, ovate, sinutelobed or toothed. Flowers white or rarely violet. Corolla funnel shaped, 7.5-12 cm. long, with 5 lobes. Capsules ovoid, 4-valved, covered with sharp slender spines. Seeds black. Flowering and fruting april to October.

Plant is frequently met with in wastelands, ardend villages, along roadsides and towns, and along roadsides upto (1000-2000) meters in the Himalayan region commonly in the tropical zones.

The leaves, flowering tops and seeds are used in medicine. The leaves and tops at the beginning and the seeds at maturity are collected.

The plant is source of hyoscyamine and fyoscine. it is used as an antispasmodic, anodyne and narcotic in tratment of branchitis, asthma and whooping cough. It is employed in various pharmaceutical formulations.

The plant contains hyoscine, hyscyamine (ditigloyls-xyropanes) tropine and pseudotrophine. The whole plant is used in skin diseases as an antiseptic.

The alcoholic extract of the entire plant possesses anticancer activity against human epidermal carcinoma of the nasopharynsx is tissue culture.

Other species of Datura which are medicinally useful and occurring in various regions of country: Datura innoxia, Datura metal Linn., and Datura suavalens.

30. Eclipta prostrata (L.) Linn. syn. Eclipta alba (L.) Hassk.

Asteraceae (Compositeae) Bhṛṅgarāja (Āyurveda)

Bhṛṅgarāja, Bhangra, Ghamra (Hindi/common names)

Annual herb, exect or prostrate, often branching and rooting at the nodes, stem and branches strigose with appressed white hairs. Leaves, sessile, variable (in breadth), usually oblong-lanceolate, sub-entire. Flowers in heads, white, solitary or 2, together (2-3) on unequal and axillary peduncles, fls. in the axil of upper leaves. ray and disc flowrs. Achenes cuneate, 2-3 mm. long, winged on the margins, no pappus. Flowering and fruting during the period from June to December.

Plant is occurring throughout India as a common weed in moist places and along drains. It is found in substropical regions in the Himalayas upto 1000 - 1700 meters herb is frequently met with in various regions in country.

Plant contains an alkaloid ecliptine and resin in high quantity. Leaves contain leucine, valine, isoleucine, phenybalmine and methiomine, glycine, glutamine, glutamic acid and cystone. Leaves are with richer content of protein. herb yields a chemical substance wedeloctone.

Whole plant, leaves and flowers or entire herb (including leaves and flowers) are used in medicine. Herb is widely used as hair tonic and employed as a major ingredient in preparing hair oils. The drug is useful in the disease of head, hair, eye, blood impurity, skin, seminal, liver, spleen and worms. It is also useful in ulcers, wounds, leucoderma, glandular affections, filiariascs, swelling, injury, tumour, syphlitic wound and other painful as well as inflammatory lesions and condtions. It is restorative (rasāyana), tonic, hypotensive, sex promotor and rejuvenating in general. The plant drug is employed in various compounds preparations.

The plant is considered to possess anticancer activity.

31. Elytraria acaulis (Linn.f.) Lindau.

syn. Tubiflora acaulis O. Kuntze.

Acanthaceae

Sahasramulā, Pādaprasarī (Āyurveda)

Patharosaga, Sasamula, Gudapasari (Hindi/common names)

Scapegerous, fibrous-rooted herb. Stems almost none. Leaves 23x9 cm., obovate, undulate, tapering below into a short, hairy petiole.

Scapes many, usually longer or as long as the leaves. Spikes 2.5-8x0.5x0.7 cm., simple or branched. flowers white, pale-coloured, much exceeding the bracts. Bracts ovate, acuminate or spine-tipped. Capsules 6-8 mm. long. Plant is flowering after the rainy season or flowering and fruiting during the period from rainy to autumn seasons.

Plant is occurring in Deccan peninsula, Ceylon and common southwards, extending northern and central Sri Lanka and to the Eastern Himalayas. it is found in the Upper Gangetic Plains, Madhya Pradesh, uttar Pradesh and Rajasthan (Marwar).

The roots, leaves and whole plant are used in medicine. the plant drug is useful in various diseases and it is administered externally as well as internally. Plant is useful in different ailments of males, females and children. In general, the plant drug is useful in fever, remittent pyrexia, colic, diarrhora, inflantile disorders, throat affections (including hoarseeness), tonsil and cold complaints by making it internal administration.

Externally it is administered in boils, abscess, tumour, boils, cyst, inflammation, gladular oedema, burns, blisters, tissue hardening, nails discolouration, wounds or ulcers and similar complaints. The roots, leaves and whole plant are ground for making into a paste are ground for making into a paste. It is externally applied to different ailments of humans. It is used in rores of cattles and animals in veterinary medicine.

The drug is considered useful as anticancer herbal agent particularly in breast cancer. This type of medicinal use is mainly based on ethno-botanical aspect of medicinal plants especially in rural and tribal regions where the plant drug is suggested to be an effective remedy for inflammatory, painful and tumourous problems of breasts. On mammary glands of females, this medicinal plants is recommended to be externally administered in conditions of cyst, abscess, boil, tumour and cancerous stage of breasts. Normally the paste of roots is made by grinding properly and the recipe is applied as an ointment or pasting over breast. The root-pieces are also rubbed on stone base (like sandal or Candana lepa) with slight water and it is pasted on breasts fuffering with different ailing condktions indicated under group of problems suggested to be treated with the plant drug which has been recommended in various other diseases. The specific application of roots obtained from plant Elytraria acaulis (Linn.f.) Lindau is considered prospective medicament of breast túmour and it opens scope for investigations in the area of breast cancer.

Elytraria acaulis Rich - A Promising Ethnobotanical Agent for Breast Tumour

Breast cancer is considered as second commonest cancer in female subjects in our country, after the cancer of cervix of uterus. Tumors of breast in women are very common and the incidence is likely to increase with the westernisation of society and other reasons. Drugs from ethnobotanical sources carry potentials as remedial agents in vrious diseases and detailed investigations have credit to contribute substantials of clinical significance. During medico-botanical exploration in tribally rich province of Madhya Pradesh, in number of ethno-botanicals with potent medicinal value were reported by author and his team C 1970-77). These records give firsthand information pertaining to a folklore phyto drug identified as Elytraria acaulis (Linn.f.) Lindau. Tribal reports claim medicinal use of this plant in treatment of abscess and tumors of breast in folk women and other ailments which have no earlier record in literature. Observations suggest possibility of its clinical potentialities in breast tumors and multi-disciplinary further studies in order to evaluate its efficacy against the tumor in general.

Excerpts are from Abstract of research papers, p.30: First National Conference on Use of Indigenous Drugs (Pandey, G.) in the Management of Cancer, February 3-6, 1988, Institute of Medical Sciences, Banaras Hindu University, Varanasi.

32. Emblica officinalis Gaertn. syn. Phyllanthus emblica L.

Euphorbiaceae

Āmalakī, Dhātrī (Sanskrit)

Anwla, Anonla (Hindi/common names)

Emblic Myrobalan, Indian Goosberry (English)

A small or moderate-sized, deciduous tree, with crooked trunk and bark light grey or greenish in colour, red inside. leaves small, very closely set in pinnate form in feathery appearance, subsessile distichous on deciduous branchlets. Flowers small, greenish-yellow, in axillary clusters. Fruits fleshy, roundish, globose, pale yellow, marked with 6 lobes or ridges; seeds angular, hard.

Plant is occurring throughout India. It is common in the mixed deciduous forests of India ascending to 1200-1350 meters in the Himalayan areas. It is often planed and under cultivation for commercial utilisation of popular fruits.

The fruit has high content of vitaminc C. Seeds contain fixed oil, essential oil and phosphates. Fruits, leaves and bark rich in tennin. Fruits contain various other chemical constituents.

The fruits are used in medicine. they are also included among dietic items in various forms. The fruits (seedless pulp) from a major drug in indigenous systems of meedicine. the drug is widely used in a number of diseases and it is a component of commonly used trio-group of myrobalans (triphalā) or Three Myrobalans. It is a restorative and rejuvenative (rasāyana) drug with preventive and curative properties. in general, the drug is useful in the diseases of digestive, respiratory and urinary systems, liver and nervous systems. The drug is therapeutically recommended in several other diseases in various forms and modes. It is employed in many formulations frequently prescribed in treatment of various ailments.

The drug is considered to possess anticancer activity. It is considered to be useful against cancer and used in treatment of cancer.

33. Erythrina arborescens Roxb.

E. variegata L.

Fabaceae (Papilionaceae)

Pāribhadra (Āyurveda)

Coral Tree (Eng.)

The plant contains erythrascine, hypaphorine, crysophorine, tetrahydrobengyl-isoquinoline and spiroamine. Locally the root decoction is useful in gout.

The alcoholic extract of the showed anticancer activity against sarcoma 180 in mice.

Small tree distributed between 1250-1700 meters in the Uttarakhanda Himalaya region and common in Garhwal at 1500 meters elevation.

Other species is occurring in the hilly region that is Erythrina suberosa Roxb.

34. Fumaria indica (Haussk.) Pugsley.

syns. Fumaria officinalis L., Fumaria parvilflora Lam.

Fumariaceae

Parpaṭa (Āyurveda)

Pittapapra, Pitpapra, Parpataka, Khetpaprha (Hindi/common names)

Annual herbs; stems diffuse, much branched, upto 60 cm. long Leaves pale green, finely divided into narrow segments. Flowers rosy-purplish, 6-8 mm. long, in terminal or leaf-opposed racemes; petals 4; the upper one spurred. Fruit globose, 1-seeded. Herbs also group as weed in wheat-barley farming fields. Flowering and fruiting during cold season.

Plant is occurring wild in upper gangetic plains, terai region of Himalayas and Nilgiri. It is commonly met with as weed herb often in wheat fields and wastelands upto, altitude of 1000 meters.

The herb contains pentatriacontane, an alkaloid 0.5%; it also contains tannin, flobefin and sugar. Ash conains potassium salts as major components.

The whole plant is used in medicine. it is useful as a good blood purifier, haemostatic, liver stimulant, anthelmintic, diaphoretic, febrifuge, stomachic, astringent, alterative, diuretic and laxative; it pacifics burning sensation and over-thrist. It is useful in skin diseases, ailments caused by blood impurities, leprosy, scrofulous cutaneous affections, liver complaints, jaundice, fever (bilary fever) gout and other diseases.

The drug is consdered to possess anticancer activity and it is useful in the treatment of cancer.

35. Glycosmis arborea (Roxb.) Dc.

syn. Glycosmis pentaphylla Corr., Limonia pentaphylla Retx.

Rutaceae

Vananimbūka, Vanya Nimbūka (Āyurveda)

Bannimbu, Chauldhua, Panal, Tarang (Hindi/common names)

Small evergreen glabrous shrub. Leaves very variable, usually 3-5-foliolate, rearely 1-foliolate. Leaflets 4-9 in. long, ovate-lanceolate ovate or obovate, obtuse, acute or acuminate, penninerved, entire or obscurely crenulate. Flowers small, white-fragrant, in erect, terminal or lateral pubescent panicles. Berry small, subglobose or somewhat compressed, white, pink or blue. Flowering and fruiting during the greater part of the year.

Plant is occurring in tropical and subtropical Himalayas from the Sutlej to Sikkim, ascending to 7000 ft. Found in Assam, peninsular India, Souther India and Karnataka.

Glycosmis mauritiana (Lank.) Tanaka. syn. Glycosmis pentaphylla Dc. is another species of the genus Glycosmis which is medicinally useful.

Medium-sized tree. leaves 5-more foliolate. leaflets ovate-lanceolate, acuminate, rounded at base, upto 12x4-6cm., coriaceous. Inflorescence brown-pubescent. Flowers white, Berry ovoid, upto 1 cm across, yellow. Flowering and fruting during the period from January to May.

Plant is occurring in Southern India, Sri Lanka; and fairly common in Upper Ghats, Karnataka.

The phytochemical studies have been conducted on the plants and various chemical constituents are recorded. Major alkaloid is arborine and other active principles isolated from plant mainly includes glycosin, arborinine, glycosminine, stigmasterol, myricyl, glycorine, glycosmine, arborinol, glycozoline, skimmianine, acridone, irboritine and other alkaloids.

The fruits, root, rook-bark, bark, leaves and whole plant are used medicinally. Plant drug is used in medicine which is used in various diseases.

The plant is useful in cough, throat complaints, rheumatism, anaemia, jaundice, fever, liver complaints, worms affection, eczema, skin complaints, inflammation, snake-bite, diarrhoea, dysentery and various other ailing. Ripe fruits are edible.

The drug is considered to be anticancer drug and it is suggested to be useful in cancer of throat.

36. Hedychium spicatum Ham. ex. Smith.

Zingiberaceae

Śaṭī (Āyurveda)

Kapurkachari, Sati (Hindi/common names)

Spiked Ginger Lily, Hedychium (English)

A robust and tall, parennial herb, upto 1.5 meters high. Rootstock thick fleshy. Leaves broadly lanceolate, 30-60 cm. long. Flowers pale yellow, fregrant, in 15-25 cm. long spikes. Capsules globose; three valves reflexed in ripe capsules; exposing the orange-red linning and numerous small seeds, enclosed in a red aril. Flowering and fruting during rainy season and onwards.

Plant is occurring in the Himalayan regions at 5000-7000 feet altitude. it is commonly wild on moist shady slapes in lower temperate regions between 1200-2000 meters elevation.

The herbs (rhizomes) contain aromatic essential oil 4%, starch (52%), carbonic acid, a glycoside and ash (4.6%).

The rhizomes are used in medicine. The drug useful as antiasthmatic anti-inflammatory expectorant, tonic, carminative, febrifuge and anti-rheumatic. it is used in respiratory disorders including eosinophilia, besides bronchitis, cough, asthma, coryza and catarrhal affections. The drug is given in heart complaint (as stimulant and cardiac), blood disorders (as blood purifier), fever, rheumatic complaints, skin affections, gastro-intestinal diseases (dyspepsia, vomiting, loss of appetite, abdominal colic and diarrhoea) and swelling. Externally the rhizomes in rheumatic conditions, flatulence, toothache, ulcers, skin complaints, foul smell (vocal) hair and head diseases.

The drug is considered to possess anticancer properties and it is suggested to be useful in cancer.

37. Hippophae rhamnoides Linn.

Elaeagnaceae

Amisa, Amila, Chuk, Tarwa (Hindi/common names)

Common Seabuckthorn (English)

Dioecious, usually spinescent shrub or small tree upto 40 ft. high, with rough brown bark. Leaves small, linear, lanceolate, covered on both sides with silvery reales. Flowers very small, greenish or yellowish, appearing with new leaves; male flowers in axillary clusters; female flowers axillary. Fruits enclosed by succulent receptacle, avoid, c. 0.25 in. long, orange yellow or scarlet. Seeds oblong, testa crustaceous shiny.

Hippophae salicifolia D.Don. is willow-like shrube. The plant is occurring almost rhroughout the temperate Himalayas. It is allied to Hippophae rhamnoides Linn.

The plants (both spices of Hippophae Linn.) are occuring in the temperate regions of the Himalayas, particularly in the river beds of drier ranges of the North-Western Himalayas at attitudes of 7,000 to 12,000 ft. altitudes.

Fruits are rich source of Vitamin C ascorbic acid 135-608, dehydro-ascorlic acid 30 mg/100 mg.). Mature fruits are rich in carotene (6-8 mg./100g.) almost half of the carrots); it also conains vitamin B. the c arotenoid pigments present in the fruit. Anthocyanin identical with peonin and flanor, iso-rhamnetin are also present. Fruits contain malic acid, citric acid, tartaric acid and traces of succinic acid, reducing sugars, pectins, tannins and mannitol. Bark contains yellow fatty oil. Twigs and leaves contain 4-5% tannin. Leaves contain cartine, abscorbic acid and some dehydro-ascorbic acid.

The fruits are acidic. They are made into a jelly with sugar and a syrup is also prepared. The drug is useful in lungs complaints and it is used in other diseases where the rich content of vitamin C becomes beneficial in human body as preventive and curative medicine.

The fruits and seed (Hippophae rhamnoides L.) are used as aphrodisiac medicine which has sexual tonic. Seeds are used in pulmonary ailments. The fruits are employed for preparing pickles sauce and similar other acidic food regimens. The bark (Hippophae salicifolic Don.) is useful for applying externally on ulcers, cuts and wounds. Fruits and seeds are commonly used as edible item of acidic and tasty plant product of hilly region. Fruits are known as stomachic, appetizer and digestive. They are considered to be promoter of disease resistance and vitalizer on account of their chemical content and properties.

38. Juglans regia Linn.

Juglandaceare

Aksota (Āyurveda)

Akhrot, Akhrut, Akhod (Hindi/common names)

Common Walnut (English)

Large deciduous trees, bark grey, bark on old stems marked by parallel furrows grey; young shoots tomentose; bark and leaves aronatic. Leaves odd-pinnate, 15-40 cm. long; leaflets 5-13, elliptic to oblong-lanceolate, usually entire; terminal leaflet largest, variable other leaflets. Flowers green unisexual. male flowers numerous, in pendulous catkins. Female flowers 1-3, clustered at the end of branches. male flowers on the shoots of previous year. Fruit drope, avoid, green, with yellow dots; pericarp leathery, aromatic. Nut wrinkled, woody 2-valved, enclosing corrugated, 4-lobed cotyledons at the single seed. Flowering and fruiting during the period from spring to autumn seasons (February to September).

Plant is occuring in Himalayan regions. It is growing wild in temperate regions usually between 2000-3000 meters. It is cultivated in hilly areas for producing edible fruit (dry fruit).

Fruit contains oxalic acid and barium. Kernel contains oil 40-45 percent, juglandin acid and ash. Immature fruit contain abscorblic acid of rich extent.

The fruit-kernels, bark, leaves and kernel oil are used in medicine. The kernel of the fruit is a medicine as well as prominent dry fruit item possessing good medicinal and nutritive values. The fruit-kernel is tonic, alternative, sexual tonic (aphrodisiac), mervine and brain tonic, demulcent, cardio-tonic anti-spasmodic, anti-rheumatic, anti-syphilitic and anthelmintic. The kernels are largely used as common dry fruit with general tonic properties.

The bark is useful as dentrific, anthelmintic, astringent, detergent and lactifuge; it is externally opplied to skin diseases. the bark is applicable to teeth but irritation is caused by presence of certain chemical substances (in excess use). The leaves are also applied (as bark use) on scabics, rores, herpes, lezeema, syphilis and scrophula. The kernel oil is useful as digestive, cholagogue, anthelmintic and usuful in various ailments. The oil is also useful for applying on leprous wounds and skin diseases.

The drug is considered to posses anticancer activity and it is useful in treatment of cancer.

39. Mucuna pruriens (L.) Dc. Syn. Mucuna prurita Hook.

Kapikacchu, Ātmaguptā, Vānarī (Āyurveda)

Kaunch, Kiwanch (Hindi/common names)

Cowhage, Cowitch (English)

Large, twinning annual; branches slender, pubescent. Leaves, 3-foliolate; leaflets membranous, 5-11x4-7.5cm broadly ovate, elliptic or rhomboid-ovate, unequal at base, acute and mucronate at apex, white pubascent beneath. Flowers dark purple, 3-35 cm. long, in 10-20cm long, drooping racemes. Pods 5-10x1.5-1.8cm; 4-6 seeded, clothed with dense, pale brown or grey irritating bristles. Seed avoid, black or dark brown marbled. Plant appears during rainy season. Flowering after rains and in antunun season and fruiting in winters to spring season.

Plant is occurring in warmer regions of India. It is growing wild in subtropical regions in the Himalayas, upto 1000 meters elevation. It is frequently net with on shrubs and bushes in serub jungles and outskirts of villages.

The seeds contain various alkaloids (alkaloidal content 0.53%) beside other chemical constituents. Seeds kernel yields an oil.

The seeds, roots and haris (bristles on pods) are used in medicine. the drug is useful in sexual and reminal disorders and general debility as a tonic. the roots and seeds are useful as nervine tonic and used in nervous disorders. the hairs or bristles are used joints worms (round worms). The drug is used as tonic, aphrodisiac, stimulant, nutritive, anthelmintic and female diseases. The seeds are employed in various compounds and drug formulations.

The drugs is considered to possess anti-cancer activity. It has been reported to be useful against cancer.

40. Phyllanthus fraternus Wesbster. Syn. Phyllanthess niruri auct.(non L.)

Euphorbiaceae

Bhūmijamalakī, Tāmalakī (Āyurveda)

Bhumiamla, Bhuianula (Hindi/common names)

Annual, much branced, ereetherb, leaf bearing branches slender, Leaves small, simples spreading (appears to be compound leaves) numerous, distichous elliptic-oblong. Flowers yellowish or creamy white, very small, axillary, hanging down below the branches. Bisesual flowers, males 1-3 and females solitary. Capsules small, globose, depressed, smooth, several scarcely or shallow lobed. Seeds minute, trigonous, brown, rounded with longitudinally ribed (regular parallel ribs on back side). Flowering and fruiting during the period from (post) rains to autumn or July to October.

Plant contains active constiuent phyllanthin, and other substances.

The whole plant is used in medicine. The drug is useful in urinary diseases, (as diuretic) gonorrhoea, leucorrhoea, chronic malarial fever, bronchitis, anaemia, dropsical disorders, diarrphoea, liver discorders, hyper acidity and poisons. It is used as restorative (resāyana) tonic and anti-ulcer drug. The herb and its different parts are used in various kinds of ulcers, wounds, tubereular ulcers, chronic ulcers offensive sores, mannary absess, and skin diseases.

The drug is considered to possess anti-cancer activity.

41. ***Picrorhiza kurroa*** **Royle ex Benth.**

Scrophulariaceae

Kaṭṭukā (Āyurveda)

Kutaki, Karu (Hindi/common names)

Picrorhiza (English)

A small react usually hairy and perennial herb, 15-25cm high, with woody rootstock. Leaves simple, spathulate, narrowed into a wingled and sheathing petiole, margins serrate. Flowers bluish-violet, in terminal racemes. Capsules avoid, acute. Flowering and fruiting during the period from summer to autumn.

Plant is occuring in the Himalayas from Kashmir to Sikkim, between the elevations of 7,000 and 13,000 feet. It grows in wild state scatteredly on moist stopes in sub-alpine and alpine regions between 3,000-4,200 meters in Uttar pradesh, Himachal Pradesh and other previous under Himalayan zone.

The root and rhizome contain two bitter glycosides picrorrhizin and kutkin, besides other chemical constitments.

The roots and rhyziomes are used in medicine. The drug is quite useful in liver disorders, hepatitis, jaundice, loss of appetite, malarial fever, oexdema, cough, asthma, bilary and skin affections. It is useful as bitter tonic. It is an effective hepatoprotective drug which is used in various diseases.

The drug is considered to possess anticancer activity. The drug has been reported to be useful in cancer.

42. Plumbago zeylanica Linn.

Plumboginaceae

Citraka (Āyurveda)

Cheeta, chitanbar, Chitrak (Hindi/common Names)

White-flowered Leadwort (English)

Perennial, sub-scandent, terate, seriate, globrous, diffuse, rambling under shrubs. Leaves ovate, entire, glabrous, base obruptily narrowed into teh petiole. Flowers white in terminal, bracteate, often branched, glandular spikes. Corolla slaver-shaped, tube-twice as long as the colysc; lobes 5. Stamens 5. Capsules oblong, patented, conained in viscid- glandular, persistant calysx. Flowering and fruiting in the period from April to November or winter season.

Plant is growing wild almost throughout India. It is found in substropical regions in the Himalayas ascending upto 1200 meters. It is fairly common in waste lands, shady places and along roadsides, Central India, Southern India and Western Peninsula and in other regions. It is also cultivated in gardens.

Roots contain a bitter crystalline, yellow, needle-like active substance, known as plumlogin, with an yield 0.91 at maximum (varying in chemical investigations depending on different factors).

The roots are used in medicine and also roots bark is also useful part for medicinal purpose. The drug is powerful stomachic and appetite promoter. It is given in gastro-intestinal complaints, haemorrhoids, worms, abdominal troubles, dysentery, loss of appltite or poor digestive power (dull stomach fire), dyspepsia, diarrhoea, skin diseases, splenic disorders, rheumatism, leucodierma (vililigo), gout and ulcers. It has irritant, vesicant, irritating and stimulating properties.

The drug is cosidered to possess anticancer activity and it is used as an ingredient or adjuvant drug in the compounds recommended in treatment of cancer. Thus the drug is included among the plant drugs sugested to be useful against cancer and its various complications.

Podophyllum hexandrum **Royle ex Camb. syn. Podophyllum** (Podophyllaceae)

emodi Wall. ex. Honig.

Erect, somewhat fleshy, perennial herbs, 15-40 cm. tall. Leaves 1-3, long petioled, palmate, deeply, 3-5 lobed. Flowers white or pink, solitary, rarely 2. Berries ovoid, 2.5-5cm. long, scarlet when ripe. Seeds many, enveloped in pulp.

Plant is in floweing and fruiting stage during the period from April to September.

Plant has regional distribution in Himachal Pradesh as follows : Temperate and alpine zone, between 2,400 - 4,500 meters. Occasionally met with as undergrowth in forests of Panarra range of Mandi forest division, and also in Kullu, Kangra, Chamba, Shimla, Kinnaur and Lahaul-Spiti division in H.P.

The rhizomes of plant are medicinally used part. They are collected in August-September during the maturity of fruits when they fully ripen.

Podophyllum emodi Wall. ex Hook. f. & thoms. An erect, glabrous, succulent herb 35-40cm high, with creeping perennial rhizome, bearing numerous root found in the inner range of the Himalayas from Kashmir to Sikkim, at altitudes of 3000-4200 meters. Leaves 2 or 3, orbicular reniform, palmate, pltate, with hood segments, flowers solitary whiter pink, cup-shaped; fruits oblong or elliptic berry, 2.5-5.0 cm diam, orange or red, containing many seeds embedded in the pulp.

43. *Podophyllum* Linn. (Berberidaceae)

A small genus of herb, distributed in the north temperate regions. three spices are reported from the Himalayan region of India of Podophyllum hexandrum Royle constitutes the source of an important pharmacopoeal drug (India Podophyllum).

The speices Podophyllum hexandrum Royle. exhibits a certain amount of variation in its botanical features. Specimens of the rent from those of the Eastern Himalayas differ from those of the North-Western Himalayas particularly in the nature of leaf-insertion. They have been classified into three or four varieties viz. var. hexandrum, var. axillaris, var. bhootnensis and var. jaeschikei.

Podophyllum emodi Wall.

Berberidaceae

Giriparpaṭa, Vanatrapusī, Vanyakarkaṭī (Āyurveda)

Bankakri, Papra, Papri (Hindi/common names)

Erect, somewhat fleshy, glabrous, succelint, perennial herbs, 15-40cm. tall. Leaves 1-3 long-petiobd, palmate, deeply 3-5-lobed. Flowers white or pink, soitary, rarely 2. Berries avoid, 2.5-5cm long, scarlet when ripe. Seeds many, enveloped in pulp. Flowering and fruiting during April to September. Rhyiomes collected during the period August-September or autumn, when the fruits attain ripening stage.

The dried rhizomes and roots of plant yields resin which is entirely used for the preparation of podophyllin from which podophyllotoxins are isolated. Besides this the resin contain quercetin, Kaempferol, astragolin and an essential oil responsible for the odour of Podophyllin. Podophyllotoxin, a and B pettairins have high potency including damage in sarcoma 37 and active in a variety of other tumours including adenocarcinoma, carcinoma and melanoma.

Plant is distributed throughout the Himalayas at an elevation of 2,500 -4,000 meters. It grows wild in alpine and temperate zones of

Himalayan region between 2,400 and 4,500 meters, and occasionally met with as undergrowth in the forests of Uttarakhand Himalaya (Garhwal and Kumaon), Himachal Pradesh (Mandi, Kulu, Kangra, Chamba, Shimla, Kinnaur, Lahul and Spiti).

The resin podophyllin obtained from rhizones is used for preparint and producing anticancer drugs e.g. etoposide and teniposide. Rhizomes are used as purgative, hepatic stimulant and indirect cholagogue.

Rhizones are collected from the inner Himalayan ranges and transported to drug market for trading. Plant species belongs to threatendd taxa facing genetic erosion, its threat status (IUCN) makes it an endangered spices due to reduction in population of over 50% in last 10 years in wild stage. Under national legistation, it falls in negative list of exports (1994) and this potential plant spices is covered by CITES and fully stands restricted.

The drug has been proved to possess anticancer activity and it is recommended therepentically for using in treatment of cancer.

The rhizome is irregular tortous, knotty, about 2-5cm. long and 1-2cm thick, somewhat flattened dorsiventrally. Upper surface is characterised by the presence of 3 or 4 cup shaped scars. colour is externally yellowish brown to larthy brown. Surface, when transeversely out, appears smooth and is irregularly circular in somewhat bitter and acrid. Powder intensely irritating to the eyes. Roots are adventitious and arise mainly from the enlarged portion of the rhizome and attain a length of about 7 cm and a thickness of 2.5 mm. Fracture of both rhizome and root is weak, brittle and even. Odour of root is slight. Taste is disagreeably bitter and acrid.

Podophyllin

Podophyllin isolated from the drug plant Podophyllum hexandrum R.&C. is considered a cholagogue, purgative, alterative, emetic and a bitter tonic. It is a drastic but slowly acting purgative producing copious watery stores; it may cause much griping and is therefore given in conjunction with belladona and hyoscyamus. It can also be used like colchicine, in cytological work because it affects spindle formation and disperses chromosomes. Owing to its cytotoxic action it is used as a paint in the treatment of soft general and other warts. Podophyllin is toxic materal strongly irritant to skin and mucous membranes. In large dose, it causes severe vomiting, diarrhoea and many result in death; exposure to its dust many cause similar symptoms.

Podophyllin is also used in veterinary medicine as a cathartic for dogs and cats. Its action on horses and cattle is variable and frequently ineffective. An ointment of podophyllin is employed to remove warts in animals and does not come in contact with the eyes.

Podophyllin and its active principles stimulate peristalsis of the isolated small intestines and of the colon of the guinea-pig, depress the isolated duodenum of rat, but cause contractions of the isolated ilaum of guinea-pig, like many other purgatives, the drug combines with serum albumin. the cardio-vascular effects of sub-lethal dose of podophyllin are reported to be relatively mild and transitory. At lethal doses, a falling respiration and muscular dystrophy were accompanied by a fall in blood pressure to shock levels. Interruption of pregnancy was produced in nice and rabbits by intravenous, subcutaneous or oral administration of non-lethal doses of podophyllotoxin. The toxin completely inhibits the larvl development of houseflies, the lowest effective concentration being 0.12 percent by weight.

Several polymorphic modification and solvates of Podophyllotoxin, with varying melting points have been obtained. In alkaline solution, it is readily converted to its C_3 eipmer picropodophyllin; the related compounds of the toxin resies likewise epimerize with alkalies to the corresponding members of the picro series. Picro Podophyllin hydrolyses with sodium hydroxide to podophyllic acid, which in turn is lactonized exclusively to the original picropodophyllin and are the alkali conversion products of podophyllotoxin. Podophyllolis believed to consist essentially of a lignan related related to podophyllotoxin, a and B-Peltaum bear the same structural relationship to each other a demethy podophyllotoxin and dehydropodophyllotoxin.

Production of drug

Most of the Indian drug is obtained at present from plants growing wild, particularly in Jammu and Kashmir, Himachal Pradesh and parts of Uttar Pradesh. Since the supply is made from inaccessible areas, the cost of collection is high and it is difficult to compete with the Amierican Podophyllum (Podophyllum peltatum) which is offered at a lower rate. Further, the Indian drug samples are not uniform in quality, as the collections are made from localities at different elevations and climatic conditions. The annual supply is at present estimated at 50-80 tonnes from the above locality which the demand is more than 100 tonnes (data pertains to 1960s decade as per records/ reports on crude drug trade).

It is stated that due to vigorous collection, to meet the increasing demand, there is a fear of depleting the natural growths, since their regeneration is slow. Steps are being advised to cultivate the plant in suitable places under forestry condtions and assure a more sustained and uniform material.

The plant drug Podophyllum or Indian Podophyllum locally known as Bankakeri (in norther India, hilly region) is highly useful in medicine. The resin podophyllin obtained from rhizomes is sued in production of modern ancicancer drugs ecoposide and teniposide. Phizomes are also useful as purgative and hepotic stimulant. It is used as an ingredient of some patent medicines (formulations) marketed as herbal or herbo-mineral drugs.

The rhizomes collected from the plants of Podophyllum hexandrum Royle ex Camb. are sold and traded in raw drug markets in India. But, the foreign trade of Podophyllum drug is banned since the plant is scheduled in negative List of Export (1994) and covered under provisions of CITES. The plant species of Podophyllum hexandrum Royle ex Camb. belongs to endgangered group of plants, its threat status (IUCN) is indangered on account of reductiton in population of 30% in last decade in wild state in the Himalayan region.

The dried shizomes and roots of Podophyllum hexandrum (Indian Podophyllum) are official in Indian Pharmacopolia and form the source of a medicinal resin. Official podophyllum contains not less than 8 percent resin, and is utilised almost entirely for the preparation of Podophyllum. Resin or Podophyllin, commonly used as a purgative. The resin content of the root and rhizomes varies with locality and the reason of collection, and on an average ranges from 7 to 15 percent. Drying of the rhizome in the sun does not appear to affect the resion content. The rhizomes collected in May has a higher resin content. Rhizome collected in November, the older rhizomes, however, yield a resin richer in podophyllotoxin. According to B.P.C., the roots form a large proportion of the Indian drug and mainly detached from the rhizome. The roots are richer in resin than the rhizomes and it has been recommended that the roots should be gathered in May when the plant is in flower.

The leaves of Podophyllum hexandrum. Royle ex Cambx yield 7-8 - 9.7 percent of resin and it has been suggested that they should form the main source of this drug in view of the slow growth of the rhizomes and roots, and the rapid depletion of the natural growth and absence of any active regeneration.

Recently, the resin podophyllin and its active principle, podophyllotoxin, have received considerable attention for their tumour necrotizing properties. Podophyllin is listed in various pharmacopolias and formularies. British Pharmacopolias recognize the dried roots and rhizomes of both Podophyllum hexandrum and the American plant Podophyllum petatum Linn. as the source of the resin drug in view of the slow growth podophyllin. The resin is extracted from the rhizome by precipitation of its alcoholic extract with slightly acidulated water. The American Podophyllum has a lower content of resin (2-8%) and its resin contain about falf the amount of podophyllotoxin as that of the Indian Podophyllum.

The plant florishes well as an undergrowth in the fir forests rich in humus and decayed organic matter. It is generally associated with species of Rhododendron, Salix, Juniperus and Viburnum, but it is also met with in open alpine meadows, where its occurrence is less frequent. The plant loves moist and shady localities situated between 2,500 and 4,000 meters.

The rhizomes and roots of the plant, which consistute the drug, are obtained entirely from wild plants growing throughout the Himalayas, especially from the Central Himalayas where they grow luxuriantly in open meadows at elevations of 3000 - 3500 meters. The undergrowth rhizomes remain dormant during winter and produce aerial shoots in April or May, depending upon the melting of snow at different altitudes and aspect. The shoots bear flower and fruit during summer and die down in November. Rhizomes which bear 3-5 aerial shoots are considered suitable for collection. the rhizomes and root are dug up in spring or autumn, cleaned dried in the sun, sifted, packed and stored in gunny bags, sometimes they are cut into cylindrical pieces and carefully dried. It is stated that rhizomes gathered in spring contain a higher resin content than those obtained in autumn. Freshly collected rhizomes are reported to contain larger quantities of active principles which are lost on prolonged storing.

In view of the inaccessible areas from where the drug is obtained and continuing demand for it both in India and abrod, attempts have been made from time to time to cultivate the plants, either from seeds or from rhizomes cuttings. Seeds under natural conditions have been found to germinate after remaining dormant for one or two years and if sown without the pulp, even failed to germinate. Preliminary treatments like soaking them in water or treatment. Preliminary treatments like soaking them in water or treating with sulphuric acid had no effect.

The seeds sown with pulp in June or July immediately after collection also remained dormant for 9-10 mouths and showed germination only in the following spring, after the melting of snow. Seeds sown in boxes, however, showed germination in 3-7 months. Seedlings so raised took a number of years to product fair-size, marketable shizomes. Propogation by rhizome cuttings, 1.0-2.5cm. In length, has also been tried. It has been found that the youngest top portions of the rhizome, bearing leafy buds gave the best results. Their growth, however, was slow and took 4-6 years to produce rhizomes suitable for exploitation.

The American podophyllum is phytochemically compared with Indian Podophyllum. The active principles, A - and B - peltatins, isolated from the former are, however, absent in Podophyllum hexandrum R. ex C. Podophyllins from the two sources are stated to differ little in their physiological activity.

Podophyllin is an amorphous powder varying in colour from light brown to greenish yellow or brownish grey, with a characteristics odour and bitter and acrid taste. On exposure to light or to temperature above 20⁰, it becomes darker in colour. Requirements of B.P. (British Pharmacoporia) for podophyllin are also recorded in respect of Podophyllin hexandrum as well as Podophyllum petatum, According to I.P. (Indian Pharmacoporia), Podophyllin (obtained from Podophyllum hexandrum) contains not less than 40 and not more than 50 percent podophyllotoyin (B.R., 1963; 625; U.S.D., 1955, 1079; I.P. 487), and other substances (sulphated ash, resin, dil, ammonia - insol matter) also shown difference.

The resins from Podophyllum peltatum and Podophyllum hexandrum can be distinguished by reacting their aleoholin solutions with aqueous potassium hydroxide, when the resin of the former does not gelatinize but that of the latter produces a stiff jelly. Another distinction is that a few drops of a strong solution of copper acetate produce a bright green colouration with the alcoholic extract of the resin from American podophyllum and a brown precipitate with that of from Indian podophyllum.

Podophyllin from Podophyllum hexandrum contains podophyllotaxin as the major active constituent, in amounts ranging from 32 to 54 percent. A number of other related compounds are their glucosides have been isolated from the resin. Lignan compounds of the Podophyllum hexandrum Royle ex Camb. follow :

Podophyllotoxin

Podophyllotoxin - B-D-glucoside

Piceropodophyllin

1-0 (BD-glucopyransyl) - Picropodophyllin

4- Demethylpodophyllotoxin

4-Demethylpodophyllotoxin, B-D-glucoside

The resin also contains queration (8%), kaempferol, astragalin (Kaempferof - 3-glucoside), an essential oil (3.7%) responsible for the odour of podophyllin, wax (8.6%) and mineral salts.

Podophyllotoxin is a lignan compund (a substance structure is based on 2-3 - dibenzyllutane) with a libile lactone ring configuration a trans (1:2) - trans (2:3) - cis (3:1)

Podophyllin has been used in the treatment of a number of disceased including cancer. It has been tried in the treatment of a various diseases particularly those characterized by warty lesions of the skin and neoplasms occurring in the resgions of the body accessible to topical therapy. It is considered the drug of choice in the treatment of condyloma ocumination because of the effectiveness, the simplicity of treatment and the absence of severe pain to the patient.

Podophyllin has been tried in tinea capitis with equivocal condition and results. It has been desirbed as an effective vermifuge, first stimulation, then paralysing and finally killing ascaris. It has given symptomatic relief in some of the allergic and inflammatory conditions of the skin. Popilloma of various sites and senile kerotoses have responded satisfactory to podophyllin.

During the last decades (1950s and 1960s) and the use of podophyllin has come into light further it has acquired special importance for its possible use in controlling some forms of cancer; the limiting factor has been the severe gastro-intestinal discomfort which follows its use in high doses. The cytotoxic effect (mitotic arrest, nucleur fragmentation, other evidence of cellular damage) of the drug is similar to that of colchicine. As a karyoplastic, it affects both dividing and non-dividing cells. The mitotic effect has been observed in skin, intestinal mucosa and tumour tissue, podophyllin. A relatively non-toxic dose levels, the peripheral blood leucocytes are reduced, the bone marrow appears hypoplastic, spleen and other lymphatic tissues are decreased in size, the adrenal cortex is depleted of lipid and marked necrosis and haemorrhage are produced in experimental tumours. The minimum effective dose (to cause appreciable damage to tumour) of podophyllin from Podophyllum hexandrum for a single subcutaneous injection in nice bearing implants of sarcoma 37, was found to be 6 mg./g. body weight.

Podophyllotixin and petation ṣ- peltatins have high potency in inducing damage in Sarcome 37 and in a variety of other tumours including adenocarcinoma, carcinoma dn melanoma. In case of nice bearing sarcoma 37, the minimum effective dose of each of the three compounds was about 24mg/g. for a single sub-cutaneous injection but several-fold higher doses were required orally. the maximum tolerated soe, in a single injection was 30-40 mg./g. for those compounds as well as podophyllin. Tumour damage was observed in general as early as 6 hours after injection. 4 - Demethypodophyllotoxin has been found to be highly active against Sarcoma 37. The other lignan compounds and their glucosides, and querectin occurring naturally in podophyllin, are much less active. the tumour damaging potency of the podophyllin compounds is said to be closely associated with their stereochemistry.

Scientific investigations for screening active constituents of the drug podophyllum and experimental studies for studying their action have been progressing since the decade of 1950s-60s and continuing further). Earlier it was observed that the mechanism of the action of podophyllin adn its active constituents on tumours was incompletely understood. It had been suggested that the necrosis is a direct consequences of a cytotoxic effect on tumour tissues; a rapid and marked reduction of the cytochrome oxidase was observed in tumour homogenes from animals treated with the podophyllin derivatives.

Another hypothesis about the mechanism of action of podophyllin and its active consituents in conditions of tumour had indicated that locus of action of the drug is the vascular system, but a number of observers have found no correlation between tumour necrotizing activity and the effect on arterial blood pressure of the drug.

Podophyllotoxin, - peltation, and ṣ- peltation have pharmacological properties similar to those of podophyllin but cause fewer undesirable or impredictable side effecs, permit precision dosage, and afford a better margin of safety when podophyllin comes in action. These crystalline products of podophyllin are commercially available. A number of derivatives of these products have been prepared for their cancer chemotherapentic studies and their methods of preparation patented. Patents have been taken for preparing stable aqueous solutions of podophyllum are commercially available. A number of derivatives of these products have been prepared for their cancer chemotherapentic studies and their methods of preparation patented. Patents have been taken for preparing stable aqueous solutions of podophyllum glucosides useful in cases of cardiac insufficiency. Amides of podophyllic and picropodophyllic acids have been found to possess very low toxicity and useful cathartic properties. Clinical trials have indicated that podophyllotoxin in useful in the treatment of Microsporium andoutini scalp injections.

The rhizomes and roots of the plant have been suggested as a source for the preparation of quercetin. The fruits are said to be edible when they ripen in June-September, they are said to be sought after and gathered by tibetan folks and other local inhabitants of inner Himalayan ranges, particularly while grazing their yak herd. No details are known about their edible properties. The fruits of Podophyllum peltatum, when ripe, have a sub-acid, sweetish, peculiar taste, and are sometimes eaten; they are also said to be preserved. When they are green or fresh, the fruits are stated to be bitter.

Podophyllum sikkimensis R. Chatterjee & Mukerjee.

Podophyllaceae

An erect glabrous herb, 15-30 cm. high, found in Sikkim. Rhizomes stout, globular, 2.3-3.0 cm x 2.0-4.0 cm. Leaves orbicular-reniform, palmate, 6-8-partite. Flowers pink, cup-shaped. Fruit an elliptic berry.

The rhizomes and roots of the plant yeild a brown resin (7.5%) possessing tumour damaging activity. The resin contains a new lignan lactone designated sikkimotoxin, 3-galactosidyl quercetin quercetin and irorhamnetin. The lactome is stated to have properties analogous to those of podophyllotoxin, and on base-calalysed eipmerization changes to iso-sikkimotoxin. A more recent investigation has raised doubt to the corectness of the proposed structure or the purity of the purity of the lactones.

The plant drug is an anticancer herbal agent. The rhizomes and roots of podophyllum sikkimensis R. Chatterjee of Mukerjee are also considered substitute of Podophyllum hexandrum Royle. syn. Podophyllum emodi Wall ex Hook. f. & Thoms, which is Indian Podophyllum belonging to the group major anticancer herbal drugs is growing obtained from plant sources naturally growing in India, particulary in the Himalayas. There are other medicinal plants which are considered to be anticancer herbal agents and they occur in the plains or non-hilly regions in India where such plants are found in wild as well as in cultivated state.

Giriparpata : An Ayurvedic drug

The taxon botanically known as Podophylum hexandrum Royle (Berberidiaceae or Polypodiaceae) is plant source of the Ayurvedic drug Giriparpata or Vanatrapusī which is known by various vernacular or regional names in different parts of country, particulary it is familiar as Vankakrhi, Paprha and some other similar names in the hilly areas under Himalayan ranges (north-west zone) where the plant grows in nature and the hill inner folks inhabiting in these hilly localities are aware about this plant and its local medicinal importance.

The plant drug Giriparpata has been defined according to the pharmacodynamics of Ayurvedic principles of pharmacology materia medica and therapiuṭics. Rasa-tikta, kaṭu; Vīrya - uṣṇa; Vipāka - kaṭu; Guṇe-laghu, rūk, tīkṣṇa and Doṣakarma-kaphapitta, especially pittasaṃsodhana.

As regards properties, action and therapeutic uses the drug Giriparpaṭa-Vanatrapusī is pittasāraka, yakrduttejaka pittarecana and pittasaṃsōdhaka; thus it is an indirect cholagogue. It is emaciating (lekhana) and irritant (kṣobhaka) and stomachic (dīpana). The drug is blood purifier (Raktaśodhana), raktaārbudanāsna auṣadhi (or anti Karkaṭārbuda drug), an anti-cancer herbal which is medicine.

The root of Giriparpaṭa is chiefly medicinally active and useful in various diseases and ailing conditions. The drug allays ailments caused by aggravation of kapha and pitta doṣa.

It is externally applied for treating skin affections (tvagvikāra) especially carmakīla; the paste of root is topically applied in this condition. The roots are emaciating and irritating as external drug.

The roots and root-extraction (podophyllin) are medicinally used and proscribed for oral administration. The drug is given in liver disorders (yakṛdvikāra) chronic constipations (jirna vibandha) and ascariasis (gaṇḍūpada krimi). Normally its extractive in 10-15 mg. dose is orally taken (for smooth or normal bowel constipation problem) and a higher dose of 15-30 mg. is recommended for internal use in case of hard bowel (krūrakoṣṭha) for countering chronic constipation as well as obstruction of portal vein. Usually the drug (in dose of 2-3 mg.) is orally administered for acting as a liver stimulant and normally it may not act as purgative.

The root-drug is internally used as stomachic, liver stimulant, cholagogue, cathartic and anthelmintic medicine. it has been pharmacologically observed that drugacts siimilar to that of colomal. It does not much increase secretion of bile, but the increased movement of investines does not absorb secreted bile.

The drug is useful in gout, rheumatism, kuṣṭha and other similar diseases. Giriparpaṭa is an ante-cancer drug which is considered to be useful against raktārbuda (blood cancer). Thus, it is included among important anti-cancer herbal agents grown in country and supported with medical texts and traditions of Indian medicine and medical practice in India.

Ol-mo-se : A potent drug in Tibetan Medicine

plant Podophyllum hexandrum Royle

Besides the modern medicine and Indian system of medicine, the Ayurveda, the drug Podophyllum, botanically is known in the tibetan medicine as ōl-mo-se. The tibetan drug ol-mo-se, the herbaceous parts of Podophyllum hexandrum Royle, is knwon in traditional Tibetan medicine for the treatment of different gynaecological diseases. The drug is also useful in other diseases. In the view of Tibetan medicine, the whole plant including the underground parts (rhizome) has medicinal utility.

The taste of the drug is considered sweet and astringent and its properties are balanced. The medicinal uses of ol-mo-se (Podophyllum) have been described in medical texts of Tibetan tradition. the drug ol-mo-se has properties of helping to improvement of assimilation and circulation of the blood and in accleration of circulation of rlung (wind), one of the main (three) principles in Tibetan medicine. It is helpful to normalise menstrual flow when it shows suffers with irregularity. Hence the drug ol-mo-se is recommended in gynaicological disorders, including the diseases of the uterus. It is also considered useful in hastuning child birth and expelling placenta during delivery under natal medicare.

Anti-cancer Herbal Agent :

Later, the plant drug in the form of rhizomes obtained from Podophyllum hexandrum Royle has been considered as a substitute for the American species Podophyllum peltatum, since the end of last century. On account of its higher content of resin, Podophyllum hexandrum fastly made replacement of American drug in the market and was further incorporated in the British and U.S. Pharmacopoeias. After the recognition of the toxic and irritant properties of the resin, both species were soon no longer admissible as a purgative. The external application as a wart-removing agent has been recommended in the pharmacopoeias. The drastic properties of the resin in the rhizome are related to the presence of the highly toxic podophyllotoxins, different arylteralin lignans which occur in varied distribution in both species i.e. Podophyllum hexandrum and Podophyllum peltatum. Since the discovery of the cytotoxic effects of the aryltetralin lignans, extensive investigations have been undertaken the chemically modified podophyllotoxins had been proved to be potent anti-tumour agents and they became anti-cancer drug in medical therapy of herbal resource in the field of oncology.

Anti-cancer Drug, Antitumor Herbal Agent and Drug for Gynaecological disorders - Plant and Drug in Tibetan Medical System

Introduction

Tibetan medicine is a traditional medical system which has been practised for centuries in Tibet and in areas influenced by Tibetan Buddhism, such as Ladakh and Sikkim in India, Nepal, Bhutan, Mongolia and those regions of the former Soviet Union which were inhabitated by Buryats and the Kalmyks. The medical heritage is based on the rGyud-bzhi, the book of the Four Tantras, whose origin can be traced back to the pre-Buddhist Bon era. The main context of the medical treatise dates from the eighth century but it has been revised and annotated throughout the year. Alothough the Tibetan materia medica is very abundant - it is comprised of many different plants, animals, minerals and even precious stones - scientific investigations concerning the identity of the drugs have been rather rare until now. this fact might be due to the long seclusion of Tibet from the outside world, the distribution of many plants and animals in remote areas at very high altitude and the reluctance of the Tibetan lamas to pass on their medical knowledge to foreigners.

The medicinal plants represent the majority of the materia medica. Several publications in western languages deal with the plant drugs used in Tibetan medicine, but very few of them were carried out by otanists or pharmacognosists. Many of the drugs which are cited in these publications are well known Indian plants, as Indian drugs have always been used in Tibetan medicine. A compilation of Tibetan drugs, mainly a literary review, was published by the Library of Tibetan Works and Archives in Dharamsala only a few years ago Pharmacognostic investigations concerning Tibetan medicinal plants, especially those which have to be collected at high altitude, are rare and the results of new scientific investigations in this field are almost solely published in Chinese or Russian at the moment.

The Institute of Pharmacognosy, Vienna, the Institute of Botany of the University of Natural Resources, Vienna, and the Tibetan Medical & Astro. Institute in Dharamsala, India, have recently entered in a cooperative alliance to undertake further investigations in the field of Tibetan medicinal plants. The main aim of this cooperation is a documentation comprising identification, morphology, distribution and ecology of the plants and description of the macroscopic and microscopic features of the drugs and their medical uses. In the course of this joint program, one of the important and frequently used plants, Podophyllum hexandrum, a drug ol-mo-se in tibetan - has been examined. Many publications can be found concerning the anatomical details of the medicinally used rhizome, but few deals with the microscopic features of the organs growing above ground.

Remarks on nomenclature and taxonomy

The name of the genus Podophyllum is derived from ancient Greek and means foot leaf. Apart from the Asian species there is one growing in America, Podphyllum peltatum, a forest plant of Altantic North America which is called May apple, becuase its fruits ripen in spring.

There are different views as to whether Podphyllum and its relatives should be given the rank of a distinct family, Podoophyllaceae, within the hierarchic system of the plant kingdom or whether they should be considered just as a subfamily, Podophylloideae, of the Berberidaceae, a family comprised of many woody, shrubby species. There are good arguments supporting botyh views. There is some confusion about the legitimate name of the drug ol-mo-se, for which the scientific names P.emodi Wall. and P.hexandrum Royle are alternately used. P.emodi was the first name given to this plant by Wallich in 1829, but it was a ñomen nudum because it was published without a description or illustration.

Royle published his P. hexandrum in 1834 together with a description. Unfortunately, he did not mention the herbaruim specimen on which his description was based. Thus it took some time until it was proven that both names refer to the same plant species. Though Wallich's name is the older one, it has to be replaced by Podophyllum hexandrum Royle, becuase it had not been published validly, i,e. not according to the rules of scientific systematics.

The species is rather variable (particularly regarding the shape of the leaves), which is no surprise if one looks at its wide range of distribution. Chartterjee distinguishes five varieties, mainly by different leaf forms and different distribution, but hara regards the characters used to distingguish between the varieties as ūnstable and variable. This opinion is shared, becuase the specimens collected by the staff of the Tibetan Medical & Astro. Institute (Dharamsala) do not fit into the Chatterjee system. A comparison of specimens in the collection of the Museum of naturla History of Vienna lead to the same conclusion. Nevertheless, the different forms seem to inhabit different areas and habitats and further investigations will have to pay attention whether particular forms are preferred for medical use or not.

The genus Dysosma, comprised of about seven Chinese species, s distinguished from Podophyllum by its peltate leaves and the number of flowers it has. Podphyllum has only one flower whereas Dysosma has several flowers arrnaged in an umbel. The name sinopodophyllum for a new genus comprised of only one species, For ōl-mo-se, P. hexandrum proposed by Ying Tsun-Shen, has not become stablished in the scientific literature outside of China and is avoided by us, becuase it could become a source of confusion.

Materials and Methods

The plant material was collected by project membes in August 1992 near Rothang-La, Himachal Pradesh, India. Voucher specimens are kept at the Institute of Botany, University of Natural Resources, Vienna, and the Institute of pharmacognosy, University of Vienna.

For macroscopic and microscopic investigations ten different samples of the various plant organs were drawn from about 250 g of the coarsely cut drug. Cuttings made by microtome and by hand were used for the description of the anatomical details. Phloroglucinol/HCL and Astrablue/Safranin were utilized as staining agents to distinguish lignified cells Microphotography was performed by Nikon Microflex AFX-DX.

Results

1. Description of the plant

In flower the erect, unbranched stem of the perennial herb is about 20cm high, later it grows up to 50cm. the size of the 2-3 alternate leaves, originating on the apex of the stem on up to 20 cm-long petiole, is about 6-20 x 4-15 cm. They are orbicular-reniform in outline and palmately divided almost to the base into three broadly elliptic or obovate acute segments with cuneate base and serrate margins, pubescent underneath. The segments range from undivided to deeply 2-3 lobed. In the early stages they are deflexed, hanging down like an umbrella. The buds are more or less terminal, later the flowers become axillary. Usually a solitary actinomorphic flower, about 2 to 5 cm in diameter, appears from May to June, consisting of (4-) 6 showy white to pinkish obovate-oblong petals and 3-6 broadly oblong sepal and usually 6 stamens, half as long as the petals. The solitary superior carpel of the bisexual plant ripens from August to September to a big ovoid fleshy fruit of up to 6x3 cm. The berry changes colour from orange to red or scarlet and bears numerous seeds which are about 2-3 mm in diameter. According to the statements in scientific floras and other printed sources the fruits are edible. The more or less horizontal rhizome is several centimeters long with thick fibrous roots reaching down more than 1m.

2. Distribution and ecology

The distribution of Podphyllum hexandrum ranges from Northeast-Afghanistan and the high mountain areas of Pakistan thoughout the Himalayas to China. As it is mainly a forest plant of the monsoon-sided slopes, in tibet it is restricted to the southernmost parts. It grows at an altitude of 2000 and 4400 m. More detailed information on the habitat of drug plant ol-mo-se is very scarce. The above mentioned altitude zone was naturally - that is before the deforesting activities of man-covered by forests. In the lower zone (2000-2500m) the forests consist of broad-leaved evergreen trees, while at higher altitude different conifers dominate, sometimes mixed with evergreen Rhododendron-tree. the upper timber-line is at around 4000 m. Where the forests are formed either by birch or juniper.

According to the laconic remarks in the floras, it is a shade-loving forest plant growing in rich human soils in coniferous forests, such as blue pine, spruce and silver fir.

According to practical experience, Podophyllum gross in birch forests, as in many areas of the Himalayas the forests.

The round fruit-stalk is 1 to 2 mm thick.

Seed:

The oval dark-red to blackish-red colored seeds are laterally applanate, 3 to 5 mm long and 2 to 3 mm broad. The surface is shiny and wrinkled. the dark coat can be distinctly differentiated from the white inner parenchyma.

Microscopic features

Leaf:

The leaf is bifacial, measuring 135 to 370 μm in width. The spongy parenchyma consists of lobed and branched cells of 10 to 40 μm large intercellular spaces which can extend to a size of about 190 μm beyond the stomata.Tthe stomata appear only in the abaxial surface of the leaf and belong to the anomocytic type with 4 to 7 (8) subsidiary cells. Occasioally two or even three stomata lie side by side without any subsidiary cells in between. Groups of stomata are found in the tips of the teeth of the leaf. As tracheids lead to and end near them, they may be associated with hydathodes. The epidermal cells of both sides are undulate sinuous, thoe of the abaxial surface are deeply curved. above the large veins the epidermal cells tend to be straight and more elongated.

The hair-covering is restricted to the margin of the spade and to the larger veins of the abaxial surface. the tube-like unicellular trichome have a club-shaped end are sometimes collapsed due to the thin cell wall. The size of the hair varies between (160-) 300 and 500 (-640) µm and the width ranges from 30 to 70 µm. In rare cases the cup-shaped end reaches a width of 115µm. Occasionally shorter hairs and even papillae can also be found. Quite often, tiny crystals of 1 to 4 µm in size and of prismatic, needle or lentil-like shape can be found in the lumen of the hairs. Similarly shaped solitary crystals of 3 to 10 µm or clustered crystals may appear in the mesophyll and along the veins. Sometimes druses, 16 to 35 µm, are gathered in groups of 2 to 7 near the veins or in the mesophyll.

The cross-section of the large veins reveals the presence of usually 3 (in rare cases 4 to 5) collateral vascular bundles arranged in a semicircle. One of the bundles is always distinctly bigger than the other ones.

Stem :

The cross-section shows an abnormal arrangement of the colateral vascular bundles, which is a known fact in this family. In contrast to the usual circular arrangement of bundles in dicotyledon, the bundles (32-76) are distributed across the stem. The majority of the differently sized bundles accumulate in the outer region of the stem forming a kind of circle, while a small number are scattered irregularly in the pith region of the stem.

The stem is bounded by an epidermis composed of elongated tangetial collenchyma cells. 5 to 8 rows of elongated parenchyma cells, scarcely showing any intercellular spaces, are situated adjacent to the epidermis. According to the varying degree of the lignification process of the parenchyma, sclerenchyma cells may appear either in the area between the outer bundles only or form a circular layer bordering the outer bundles only or form a ciruclar layer bordering the outer parenchyma tissue. the sclerenchyma cells show a wide lumen and reach a diameter of 8 to 60µm and a length of 250 to 700 µm. When present the cirulcar sclerenchyma layer merges above the bundles with a tangential band or a hood of long, slightly thicker, pitted fibres. This layer of fibre which always hoods the phloem of the vascular bundle is 1 to 11 rows high. the bundles may not only be hooded by fibre, but can also be encircled by them. the diameter of the fibres varies between 5 to 40 (54) µm, the length of the fibres is upto about 1400 µm. The xylem is characterized by vessels showing different wall thickening, annular, helical, scalariform thickening and also pitting. The width of the tracheary elements ranges from 10 to 54 (62 (µm. The pith tissue is composed of parenchyma cells which may occasionally be pited. Crystal druses can be found in all parenchyma cells of the stem, reaching a size of (14-) 30 to 40 (-58) µm. Starch grains are not present.

Fruit :

The exocarp is composed of tangential collenchyma cells showing in the cross-section a rectangular shape and a size of usualy 20 to 50 µm by 20 to 30 µm. Stomata of the anomocytic type may be present. The first 5 to 6 rows of the mesocarp cells are distinctly bigger and exhbit little tangential collenchyma. the following thin-walled cells of the inner part of the pulp are either collapsed or destroyed. Vessels with helical thickening and druses, 22 to 40(-54) µm, can be found.

Fruit-stalk:

The epidermis consists of elongated cells with lamellar collenchyma thickening. Adjacent to the epidermis, the cortex is formed by 4 to 11 rows of parenchyma cells occasionally showing intercellular spaces. The cross-section reveals a biserial circular arrangement of vascular bundles. The outer circle contains 11 to 18 (-24) bundles, the inner one (3-) 5 to 7 (-9) usually bigger bundles. Each bundles has a layer of fibre hooding the phloem or is surrounded by a sheath of fibre. The medullary rays and the pith are composed of parenchyma cells separated by angular intercellular spaces. A hollow pith may be present. Druses measuring usually 15 to 40 µm can be found. Due to the characteristic grouping of the vascular bundles, the fruit-stalk can easily be distinguished from the stem by its anatomical features.

Seed:

Three distinct layers can be distinguished in the seed coat. the bounding layer is composed of one rows of elongated, lignified cells which in the cross-section display a palisade-like shape and a remarkably thickened outer cell wall. The cells are on the average (20-)40 to 40µm broad and 80 to 155 µm high; the outer wall is 6 to 13 µm thick. The size of the palisade cells changes depending on its position int eh seed; broader and higher palisades are present near the micropyle. the characteristic palisade cells are followed by a broad band of parenchyma which represents a large part of the testa tissue. The innermost layer of the testa is developed as a row of brownish-coloured, flat cells, 10 to 15 µm high, each one containing several solitary crystals. The crystals are rhomboidal and measure between 2 and 9 µm. The nutritive tissue and the cotyledons consist of parenchyma cells. Starch grains are not present.

Summary

The Tibetan drug ol-mo-sȩ consists of the dried, coarsely cut above-ground parts of the plant, the leaves, stems, fruits and seeds. The leaves are light green to brownish-green, show a digitately parted blade and a serrate to dentate, slightly ciliate margin. The stem is yellow to light brown, grooved and glabrous. Frequently, parts of the reddish fruit with the embeded dark seeds can be found. The drug has no characteristic odour, the taste of the stems and leaves is slightly bitter, the fruit is sweet and the seeds are astringent.

Microscopic characteristics of the leaf are the tube-like, unicellular, thin walled, 300 to 500 µm long trichomes in the margin and on the larger veins of the abaxial surface. Unusual groupings of the stomata which occur in paris or in groups of three without any subsidiary cell in between can be seen. Occasionally, shorter hair (>160µm) and papillae are found. Crystals may appear as tiny needles in the hairs and as solitary crystals (3 to 19 µm) or clustered crystals in the mesophyll and along the veins. the large veins usually bear 3 collateral vascular bundles, each one hooded or surrounded by a sheath of long fibres. A layer of sclerenchyma cells may appear either in the inner part of the cortex or between the outer bundles. Crystal druses (30 to 40 µm) can be found in all parenchyma cells. The fruit wall consists mainly of parenchyma tissue, occasionally with druses (22 to 40 µm). The fruit stalk can be distinguished from the stem by the biserial arrangement of the vascular bundles. the seed coat is composed of a bounding layer of prominent lignified, thick-walled palisade-like cells, a parenchyma tissue and an inner row of brownish cells, each one containing several solitary crystals (2 to 9 μm). Starch grains are not present in the nutritive tissue.

Use in Tibetan medicine

In one of the still acknowledged famous Tibetan medical books of the 18th century, the Dri Med shel gong and dri med shel phreng, ōl-mo-se is mentioned as an important medicinal drug which cures womens disorders and blood disorders and which is applied externally in certain cases of skin diseases. In this treatise various opinion of older medical books and opinions of famous lamas are cited and a short description of the plant is given. The botanical description reveals a good observation of significant morphological characteristics and even gives some information on the site. The plant is described as growing in the forests, with a hard root and many small ones, with big lea.es and a long stem, with a beautiful red coloured flower[c] and fruit in the shape of cattles testicles, resembling a blood-filled bulge in colour. The taste of the root is bitter and pungent, that of the leaf bitter and astringent, while the fruit is sweet. The seeds are red to brown in colour. In this monograph, a warning is even given to avoid excessive external application of the powdered drug, as serious blisters may arise. According to this medical treatise, the whole plant, including the underground organs, was in medical use at that time.

Regarding the opinion of the Tibetan doctors in Dharmsala, the taste of the drug is considered sweet and astringent and its properties balanced. The use of ōl-mo-se are described as follows: ōl-mo-se helps to improve the assimilation and circulation of the blood, accelerates the circulation of rlung, corrects menstrual irregularity and is used for the treatment of gynaecological diseases, including diseases of the uterus. It is also used to clear out the placenta and to ease child birth.

Use of Podophyllum species in western medicine

The rhizomes of Podophyllum hexandrum Royle have been known in Western medicine as a substitute for the American species P. peltatum since the end of the last century. Due to its higher amount of resin, P.hexandrum quickly replaced the American drug on the market and was even accepted in the British and US Pharmacopoeias. After having recognised the toxic and irritant properties of the resin, both species were soon no longer admissible as a purgative. At present only external appliction as a wart-removing agent is recommended in the pharmacopoeias. The drastic properties of the reisn in the rhizome are related to the presence of the highly toxic podophyllotoxins, different aryltertralin lignans which occur in varied distribution in both species. Since the discovery of the cytotoxic effects of the aryltertralin lignans, extensive investigations have been undertaken. Chemically modified podophylotoxins proved to be potent anti-tumor agents and were introduced into medical therapy. The herbaceous parts of the plant have never given rise to the same interest as the rhizome. A few years ago investigations of the above ground parts of P.peltatum revealed the presence of 3 new anti-fungal substances, the di-hydro2-pyrone derivatives Podoblastin A,B, and C.(kletter, ch. sman-rTsis, vol.1, No.1, 1995, 1-23).

44. Panica granatum Linn.

Punicaceae

Dāḍima (Āyurveda)

Anar (Hindi/common names)

Pomegranate (English)

Large deciduous shrubs or small trees with smooth and dark grey bark; branchelets armed with small, axillary terminal the of Leaves opposite, 2-8 cm. long, oblong or obovate, oblong-lançeola and in varying shape, entire, bright green. Flowers scarlet red, sometimes yellow, solitary or together (2-4). Fruits globose, crowned by persistent calyx-lobes; rind coriaceous, woody, interior septate with membranous wall of the carpels, each carpel containing numerous seeds. Seeds angular from mutual pressure, seeds with a watery coat containing pink juice, seed with fleshy testa of red, pink or whitish colour. Flowering and fruiting during the period from summers to autumn.

Plant is growing wild in warm valleys and outer hills of the Himalayas between 900 and 1800 meters. It is planted throughout India, cultivated commonly for edible fruits (tasty seeds of sweet with acidity).

The seeds, fruit pericarp (rind), stem (stem-bark) and roots (root-bark) etc. have chemically been screened and their chemical profile shows various contents in different parts. Tannin is a common content which is found various in most of the part premominantly in fruit rind, stem bark, root bark and leaves. The edible portion (68%) of pomegranates contain fat, protein, fibres, other carbohydrates, mineral matters, calcium, magnesium, oxalic acid, phosphorous, iron, sodium, potassium, copper, sulphur, chlorine, caroteme, thiamine, riboflavin, nicotinic acid and vitamin C (14mg./100g.). Fruit is a good source of iron but is poor in calcium, and a fair source of iron. Fruit contains 0.27 percent of pectin (as calcium pectate). Bark stem and roots contain a number of alkaloids belonging to the pyridine group. The alkaloids have their tannates; and d.- mannitol occurs obundantly in stem bark and in lesser amounts in root bark, seeds and leaves. Friedelin and betulic acid are reported in bark, betulic and ursolic acids in the leaves, and ursolic acidy in the fruit rind. Leaves of young plants contain an unstable alkaloid.

The fruits, seeds (dried seeds as ānardana or bihidana) rind, stem, roots, flowers and leaves are medicinally useful; and the fruits (seeds) are deliciously used as common edible fruit possessing high medicinal and nutritive value. The drug, is cardiac, tonic, refrigerant, stomachic, astringent, anthelmintic and laxative; and it enriches blood.

The extracts of different parts of the tree exhibited antibiotic activity. Extracts of the whole fruit have been found highly antimicrobially active; they are also proved to be very effective against intestinal pathogenic bacilli. The alcoholic extract of the intestinal root fruit rind and antimicrobial activity. Aquaous extract of the root has also been found to possess potent antimicrobial activity. The leaves and fruits gave a positive haemoloysis test. Extracts of the fruit rind (at a concentration of (og./litre) are reported to show like other tannin-bearing plants, positive inhibition against, certain fungi.

The drug is considered to possess anticancer activities and useful in cancer.

45. Rubia cordifolia Linn.

Rubiacear

Manjiṣṭhā (Āyurveda)

Manjitha, Manjeetha (Hindi/common names)

Indian Madder, Dyers Madder (English)

Perennial climbing herbs; stems and branches 4-angles minutely prickly. Leaves in whorl of 4 long-stalked, ovate, cordate, long-pointed, nerves and margins prickly. Flowers small, dark-red or pinkish-brown, in numerous small cymes, forming large bracteate panicles. corolla 5-lobed. Stamens 5. Fruits succulent, globose or slightly, 2-lobed, black; seeds two. Flowering and fruiting during, the period from June to September.

Plant is occurring in substropical and temperate regions in the Himalayas upto 2,400 meters elevation.

The roots used in medicine. Roots are astringent, alterative, deobstruent and tonic. the drug is used in the treatment of paralysis, jaundice, fever, obstruction in urinary passages, menstrual disorders, inflammatory condition of the chest and skin diseases. Being an important drug of indigenous system of medcine, the drug is employed in various compound formulations.

The roots of the plant have been reported to possess anticancer activity. Roots are considered to be useful in treatment of cancer in various forms.

The roots are collected during winter season. Roots in dried state from the crude drug material of Majeeth marketed in raw drug trade.

46. Semecarpus anacardium Linn.

Bhallātaka (Āyurveda)

Bhilawa (Hindi/common name)

Marking Nut (English)

Moderate sized tree. Leaves 18-60 x 10-30 cm., abovate-oblong, rounded at the apex, coriaceous; glabrous above, ashy grey, or half and more less pubescent beneath, sometimes shortly aruricled; main nerves 15-25 pairs marking a large angle with the costs patioles 1.2-3.8 cm long. Flowers greenish-white, subsessile; fascicled in pubescent panicles shorter than the male pedicels short, Drupes 2.5 cm. long, obliquely, ovoid or oblong, smooth and shining, black when ripe, seated on a fleshy orange-red cup, receptacle or hypocarp short 2 cm. long, smooth and yellow when ripe. Flowering and fruiting during the period from December to June.

Plant is distributed in the hotter parts of India nd also in the Himalayas from ascending to 1,100 meters elevation. It is growing in sub-Himalayan tract and outer hills; Central India, Assam and western penisula.

The fruit contains anacardiac acid, cardol, catechol, anacardol and a fixed oil, samecarpol and bhilawanol. The oil of fruit is blistering and yeild of oil is 32 percent. Fruit kernels contain a little quantity sweet oil.

The fruits are used in medicine. The therapentic administration of only purified fruit (śodhitā or śuddha bhallātaka) is recommended in Indian medicine, where it is used in various diseases. The drug is useful in ascites, vāta and kapha roga, piles, dysentery, tumours, fevers, loss of appetite, urinary discharge; it is given in asthama, insanity, worms, leprosy, bronchitis, inflammation syphilis, dyspcpsia, nervous debility, neuralgia, skin diseases, paralysis, leucoderma, snake-bite, veneral diseases and sexual importency. It is rasāyana (promotive and aphrodisiac) drug.

The drug is considered to possess anticancer activity and it is therapeutically used in treatment of tumour (arbuda) and its various kinds (cancer) in different forms and as an ingredient in certain formulations recommended in cancer therapy.

The drug Guggulu (purified) prominently is used for treatment of cancer and generally it is found to be major component of various compound formulations which are frequently prescribed for treating cancer in idigenous system of medicine recommending use of guggulu (olo-gum resin of Commiphora mukul) in management of cancer. Some classical formulations (sāstriya yoga) are worthmentioning as follow:

A. 1. Kāncanāara guggulu
   2. Pancatikta ghrta guggulu
   3. Vranāri guggulu
   4. Kaiśora guggulu
   5. Triphalā guggulu

6. Pṅcavinśati guggulu
7. Yogarāja guggulu
8. Other guggula yogāah (compounds)

B. 1. Arogyavardhini vaṭī
2. Candraprabhāvatī
3. Other formulations.

47. Saussurea costus (Falc.) Lipsch.

Syn. Saussurea lappa (Decne) Sch-Bip.

Asteraceae (Compositeae)

Kuṣṭha (Āyurveda)

Kuth (Hindi/common names)

Costus, Kuth (English)

A tall, robust, pubescent herbs, 1.2-2 meters high. Leaves membranous, irregularly toothed based ones very large triangular with a long winged stalk; stem leaves smaller, sessile or stalked, with a narrow auricled base. Heads purple, sessile, axillary or in terminal clusters. Achenes compressed curved upwards. Pappus brown. Flowering and fruiting in June-September.

Plant is occurring in the Himalayan regions of Kashmir, Himachal Pradesh and Uttar Pradesh. It is also cultivated in sub-alpine, cold and humid region of the hilly regions.

The roots contain resinoid (6%), intense odorous oil (1.5%), saussurine 0.05%, tannin, inuline 18%, a fixed oil and other substances. Leaves contain little alkaloidal principle and sterol. Roots yield essential oil containing various odorous substances.

The roots are used in medicine. The drug is stimulant, stomachinc, tonic, antifungal, antiseptic, aromatic, astringent, sedative and carminative. It is useful as spasmodic, alternative, aphrodisiac and, antirheumatic and antidermatitis. The drug is blood purifier, diaphoretic and restorative (rasāyana). It is analgesic and germicidal. Besides neurological disorders, it is used in various diseases as an effective and valuable drug in medicine. Biological studies find alcoholic extract as strong antifungal action. It has increased value. The drug is considered to possess anticancer properties and it is recommended to be useful in treatment of cancer.

48. Taxus wallichiana Zucc.

Taxus wallichiana. zucc. Syn. Taxus baccata auct. (non L.)

Sthouṇeyaka, Tālīśa (Ayurveda)

Talispatra, Birmi, Taxus, Thuner (Hindi/common names)

Himalayan few (English)

Small or medium-sized, evergreen trees; branches horizontal. Leaves 2.5-3.8 cm. long, linear, flattened, distinchous, spines-tipped, beneath, aromatic dry. Male cones small, globular. Female conces consisting of a solitary ovule, surrounded at the base by a cup-shaped disc, which enlarges and becomes succulent and bright red at maturity. Seed olive green. Flowering and fruiting during the period from march-May to September-November.

Plant is occurring wild in evergreen and coniferous forests of temperate Himalayas. It is found in various Himalayan regions falling between 2800 and 4000 meters elevation. Trees grow in hilly forests of Uttar Pradesh, Jammu & Kashmir, Himachal Pradesh, Meghalaya, and West Bengal etc. in India.

The bark and leaves mainly stem bark are source of 10-deacetyl-baccatin III (DAB III) which is chemically converted into taxol, a potent anticancer drug. It is used in treatment of ovarian and breast cancer. The needles also contain betuloside which is a potent liver protecting drug. Several other consitutuents have been isolated from different parts of plant.

The bark and leaves are medicinally used. Leaves are used in indigenous sysstem of medicine. It is botanical source of drug Sthouneyaka as well as a substitute or adulterant of the drug Tālīśa: it is considered one of the plant sources for Talisa or Talispatra The drug is an important medicine for cough, bronchitis and asthma and allied complaints of respiratory system.

The plant falls under category of endangered species due to raduction in population (over 50% in last 10 years in wild state). The collection of plant material has been reported to be banned (Uttarakhand Himalaya, U.P.) and it has consequently been included in the negative list of export (1994) of medicinal plants growing wild, collected and traded from India.

49. Terminalia bellirica (Gaertn.) Roxb.

Combretaceae

Bibhitaka (Āyurveda)

Bahera, Baherha (Hindi/common names)

Beleic Myrobalans (English)

Medium-size or large deciduous trees, with thick and dark-green or bluish-grey bark, trees generally conspicous. Leaves large, broadly-elliptic or elliptic-obovate, rounded or rarely sub-acute or shortly acuminate; leaves crowded lowards end of branches, lvs. greyish-green in colour pale beneath. Flowers small, greenish-yellow, in single slender spickes, with an offensive odour. Fruit drupe 2-3 cm. long, ovoid or ellipsoid, grey-velvety, grey, velvety, thick, hard, obsurely 5-angled when dried; fruits with hard and pentagonal stone. Flowering and fruiting in the period from spring to autumn season.

Plant occurring throughout the deciduous forests in India and also planted along roadside. It also ascends in hilly regions upto about 3,000 feet. in sub-tropical regions in open deciduous forests and roadsides near plantations (upto 1000 meters) and sporadic in warm valleys.

The fruits contain 17% tannin. Seeds kernal contain 25% fixed oil. Fruits also contain gall-tannic acid, colouring matter and resin. Seeds yield greenish-yellow oil.

The fruits (stoneless) are mainly used in medicine. The drug is quote useful as expectorant, laxative, tonic and astringent. Fruits are used in various forms and modes in several diseases especially in treatment of diseases of respiratory, digestive and also nervous system, alongwith various other diseases of different systems and organs. The drug is much used is cough, asthma, coryza, constipation, eye diseases, piles, dyspepsia, throat affections, opthalmia, diarrhoea and haemorrhages. Externally the ponder of dried fruit is applied on cut, bruises, wounds for astringent and haemostatic action and the paste is also applied an wound and in eye ointment (conjunctivitis).

The fruits are major component of Triphalā (consisting three drugs viz. Harītakī, Bibhitaka and Āmalakī) carrying classical base of Indian medicine. The drug is valuable and employed in a number of medicinal preparations or compounds used in medical system.

The drug is considered to be useful in treatment of cancer.

50. Terminalia chebula (Gaertn.) Retz.

Combrataceae

Harītakī (Āyurveda)

Haroor, Harad, Haritaki, Harra (Hindi/common names)

Chebulic Myrobalan (English)

A medium-sized or large deciduous tree. Leaves glabrous or nearby so at maturity, distant, alternate or sub-opposite, broadly elliptic - oblong, rounded or cordate at base, patiole 2 (or more) - gland dotted 3 penninerved. Flowers hermaphrodite, dull-white yellow in spikes, yellowish-green, at the end of branches. Fruit drupe, 2-4 cm. long, obovoid, yellowish-green, pendulous, glabrous, 5-angled or ribed (more or less) when dry, acute, bony, hard nut, very thick. Flowering in April-June and fruiting in July-March.

Plant is occurring throughout greater part of India, specially in central, northern and southern India and its occurrence assending in outer Himalaya upto 5000-6000 feet elevation.

Fruits contain tannin upto 30% chebulinic acid, gallic acid, resin and other substances - including mucilaginous and colouring matter. It contain also chebulagic acid, corilagin, aminos acids and other constituents in lesser quantity. Seeds kernel yeilds an oil yellow in colour (36.4%).

The fruits are used in medicine. the drug enjoys a cadre of highly valuable among major drugs of Indian medicine. The drug is alterative and rejuvenation or restorative (rasāyana) and laxatives besides stomachic, astringent, tonic, carmivative and expectorant. It possess various medicinal properties and it is used in large number of diseases including tumour, cysts in various forms and modes. It is employed in a number of pharmaceutical preparations of formulations. The drug is also applied externally. The fruits are components of three myrobalans or Triphalā (comprising the fruits of Terminalia chebula, Terminalia bellirica and Emblica officinalis, known as Haritakī, Bibhītaka and Āmalakī respectively).

The drug is considered to possess anticancer properties and useful in the management of cancer.

51. Tinospora cordifolia (Willd.) Hook.f. & Th.

Menispermaceae

Guḍūcī (Āyurveda)

Giloy, Gurch, Gurch, Gulancha (Hindi/common names)

Large deciduous, glaucous, glabrous twiners, climbers with succulent, corky grooved stems, bark light, grey, papery, branches bending down slender pendulous Fleshy roots, terete, striate, with tubercled, pale sometimes shining or glaucous bark. Leaves membranous, 7-9-nerved 5-10 cm., roundish, subdeltoid, cordate with a broad sinus and large basal lobes, obtuse, more or less cuspidate, reticulately veined. Flowers small, greenish-yellow, dioecious, in racemes, on nodes of the old stems. Male and female flowers. racemes rather lax, 5 cm. long elongating and finally often longer than the leaves, axillary, terminal or from the old wood. Carpels, drupes ovoid, red when ripe, fleshy, larger pea-size; stone broadly ellipsoid. Flowering and fruiting in March-June.

Plant is occurring throughout warm regions in India. Large climbers are often found on tree and shrubes etc. mostly in tropical regions. It grows in deciduous forests of substropical regions in warm valleys in the Himalayan zones, generally ascending upto 1000 metes.

Plant contains berberine, bitter substance, starch and a neutral substance. Fresh stems give crude gilon and gilonin, and also some other substances.

The stem is used in medicine and watery extract 3 guḍūcī satva or sat giloy), in the form of white powdder) is frequently used in therapeusis. The drug is alterative antibilary antiperiodic, anthelmintic, antiarthritic, aphrodisiac, blood-purifier, bittertonic, stomachic and anti-rheumatic (gout); it is a restroative (rasāyana) drug. It is therapentically used in several diseases, being very important drug of Indian medicine.

The drug is considered to possess anticancer activity and cancer protective properties, it is found to be immunomodulator, immunity promoter enhencing disease resistance. It is considered imnunostimulant, hepatoprotective and antioxidant herbal agent.

52. Urtica dioica Linn.

Urticaneae

Stinging Nettla common stinging Nettle (Eng.)

Vṛścikapatrī, histamine/and 5-hydroxytryptamine and a histamine liberating enzyme is also present. It has high percentage of proteins.

The drug is recommended for the treatment of haemotptysis and other haemorrhages. Leaf infusion is used in wounds. Roots, leaves and, seeds and leafy herb are used medicinally.

Small herb distributed between the elevation of 200 - 3200 meters. Temperate zones regin falling between the elevation of 1000 to 2500 meters in forests shrubheries. It grows abundantly as commonly as itching plant in various regions of Western Himalayas at elevation of about 5000 ft. and above.

Stinging herbaceous perennial, with opposite ovate to lanceolate, coarsely toothed leaves, and tiny green flowers in long axillary, tassel-like hanging or spreading clusters not longer than the leaves. Flowers unsexual, on different plant; male flowers with 4-ovate perianth-segments with 4-stamens; female flowers with subequal segments, stigma like a tuft of hairs. Leaves 5-10 cm. with a pair of elliptic stipules at the base. Stem rather robust, grooved, 80-175 cm. Achenes flattened encircled by the persistent perianth. Flowering and fruiting in August - September and onwards.

53. Viola pilosa Blume. Syn. Viola serpens Wall ex Ging.

Violaceae

Vanapsikā, Vanapuṣpā (Āyurveda)

Banfasha, Gul Balafsha (Hindi/common names)

Prostrate to subprostrate herbs; stems or stolons usually long, leafy. Leaves ovate to deltoid, shallowly cordate at base, 1.5-8x1-6 cm., serrate; petiole 2-10 cm. long; stipules ovate-acuminate, subentire to dentate. Flowers white or pale violet; peduncles 3-8cm. long, piolose; styles subclavate, subtruncate and shortly beaked at apex, Capsules ellipsoid, glaucous. Flowering and fruiting almost through out the year, particularly March-July.

Plant is commonly occurring in moist slopes in temperate forests and meadows, between 1,200-3x000 meters in Himalayan regions.

The whole plant (burg banofsha) and specifically flowers (gul banfsha) are used in medicine. The herb is diaphoretic, antiphyretic and effective febrifuge. Particularly the flowers are excellent expectorant and commonly given in ough, cold and fever alongwith sore throat and other throat affections. The drug is also useful in kidney problems, infantile complaints, liver disorders and some other ailments.

The drug is censidered to possess anticancer activity and properties as cancer protective effect and curative qualities.

The crude drug, generally collected green herbs as well as flowers, during spring to summers, forms dried aerial parts and the flowers, is markted in raw drug trade. some allied species of Viola are also collected, administured and used, such as Viola canescens Wall and others.

54. Vitis vinifera Linn.

Vitaceae

Draākṣā (Āyurveda)

Angur, Datch (Hindi/common names)

Grape (English)

Large deciduous climber grape vine with long and bifid tendrils. Leaves 7.5-15cm. long, orbicular-cordate, more or less deeply (3-)5-lobed, margin toothed. Inflorescence leaf-opposed of panicled cymes. Flowers green. berry variable in size, bluish black or greenish. Seeds 2-4, pear-shaped. Barries in lunches. Flowering and fruiting in various seasons; August-September to December-January.

Plant is cultivated in various regions, particularly north-western India. It is planted in houses and gardens; it is under commercial farming for edible grape gruits.

The fruit juice contains malic, trartaric and racemic acid, and it contains glucose and other substances. Fruits contain various other acids (sulphuric, salisylic and phosphoric acids), potassium, magnesium, sodium, iron and other minersls. Fruits contain 15 I.U. vitamin A, meacin 3 mg., rivoflavin 10 and vitamin C 15 mg (Vitamin B complex and Vitaminc C)

The fruits are mainly used in medicine as other parts also medicinal and they are commonly edible and delicious grape-fruit (berries) of sweet taste (ripe) and juicy. The fruits are tonic, cardiac, cooling, refrigerant, laxative, appetiser, demulcent diuretic, astringent and aphrodisiac. Fruits are useful in diseases of heart, lungs, liver, kidney, throat, stomach, intestines, spleen and other organs and systems. It is useful in general debility as well as in consumption and as restorative and vitalizer (rasāyana - jivaniya).

The fruits are considered to possess anticancer activity. Grapes (ripe and sweet fruits) have been reported to be useful in treatment of cancer besides its cancer protective properties. The effeicacy of fruits have therapeutically been indicated in management of cancer. There is reference of grape cure for cancer (About Grape Cure by V. Shaikil and other works by J. Bandit giving details of cancer treatment by grape fruits) and also other parts of medicinal plant. Accordingly, the cancer patient is firstly advised for fast of three days, before grape therapy for cancer, and only boiled water is allowed. The juice of grapes is given as drink for a week by restricting any other food intake. Enema once in evening is applied for evacuation. Druing the day, about 250 gms. grapes are given thrice (e.g. morning, noon and evening) by continuing for a month. The butter milk or fat free cured liquid (takra: Sanskrit) is given twice (e.g. forenoon and afternoon). Other food or diet are normally restricted. In addition, the branches of grape vine are also suggested for formentation in cases of externally affected body parts (cancer lesions). A poultice of pericarp (fruit covering) is also recommended in such condition (wherever external application is required).

It has been discussed about grape therapy of cancer that the intake of grapes lights against carcinogens and expets them out or exeretes through urine as urination may increase during the treatment of cancer. In case the pain in abdomen and rectal (and) burning sensation, the intake of grapes may continue as these sysptones are likely to subside after sometime. The motion (passing stool) can also be disturbed, and later normal evacuation.

Thus, the therapy of grapes coupled with fasting (npavāsa-angur or drākṣārasa kalpa) has been appreciably recommended in management of cancer. Alongiwth the juice of grapes, only the juice of Emblica officinalis Gaertn. or Emblic Myrobalans (āmalakī-anwla) can be given and also the juice of some suitable seasonal fruits and vegetables specially in case of burning, pain and uneasiness in abdomen of patient.

The use of grapes has been appreciated for its efficiency in various ways due to specific potentiantialities actively suitable in combating cancer.

55. Vitex negundo Linn.

Verbenaceae

Nirguṇḍī, Sinduvāra (Āyurveda)

Samhalu, Samalu, Nirgundi, Meurhi (Hindi/common names)

Five-leaved chaste (English)

Large shrubs, with spreading branches. Leaves opposite, digitately 3-5 foliolate; petiole 2.5-5cm. long; leaflats 5-15cm. long, lanceolate, entire, crenate or coarsely serrate, nearly glabrous above, covered with fine white tomentum beneath. Flowers blue or lavender, in large terminal paincles; coralla 2-lipped, 5-lobed; stamens 4, exerted. Fruits 5mm in diam., globose, black when ripe; exocarp succulent; endocarp bony, narmally 4-celled. Flowering and fruiting in spring-summers and winter season.

Plant is occurring throughout India especially in warm regions. it grows wild in the sub-tropical regions in the Himalayas according to 200 meters. Plant is common in hedges along roadsides, rivers, canals and other localities (including warm valleys in hilly regions). It is also planted.

The leaves contain aromatic volatile oil and resinous substance. Fruits contain tannin, carbonic acid, malic acid and an alkaloid and colouring matter.

The leaves, root, flowers and fruits (seeds) are used in medicine. The drug is effectively used as anti-inflammatory, antiseptic, analgesic and wound healing drug. It is useful in rheumatic disorders and various ailments characterised by inflammation and pain. The drug is used in ulcers, sprains, wounds, sinus, scabics, itching, dermatitis, sciatica, fever, cough, coryza, pleurisy, eye and lear diseases and other various ailments. It is also restorative (rasāyana) and useful in general debility. The drug is administered both externally and internally.

The drug is considered to possess anticancer properties and useful in treatment of cancer.

Withania somnifera (L.) Dunal.

Solanaceae

Aśvagandhā (Āyurveda)

Asagandh, Asvagandha (Hindi/common names)

Winter Cherry (English)

Branched erect undershrub, upto 1.5 m. high; branches terete, clothed with stellate tomentum. Leaves ovate, entire, 7-15cm. long, petiole upto 2.5 cm. long. Flowers greenish or lurid-yellow, in sessile or subsessile, umbelllate cymes. Berries red, globose, smooth, about 6mm. diam., enclosed in the much enlarged, inflated and membranous, somewhat 5-angled, pubescent calyx. Seeds yellow or palebrown, subreniform, wrinked. Flowering and fruiting almost throughout the year specially from rainy season to autumn season.

Plant is occurring in drier regions of India and it is grown in wild state almost throughout country ascending upto 5000 ft. elevation or substropical regions upto 1200 meters. It is frequently found in wastelands (rather dirty places and waste spots) in drier and warm regions in central India, Karnataka, Andhra Pradesh, Rajasthan, Tamilnadu, and West Bengal and other regions in India.

The roots of plant contain a volatile oil and an alkaloid withoniol. they also contain a crystalline alkaloid somniferin and phytosterol and active substances. Leaves and stemss (water soluble extracts) also contain almost same or various chemical constituents in addition to potassium nitrate. The roots, in general, yeild alkaloidal content 0.13%-0.31% in total, which includes about 13 or more alkaloids and derivatives.

The roots are used in medicine. the drug is stimulant, alterative, tonic, aphrodisiac, diuretic, analgesic, doeobstruent and hypotensive.

It is a rasāyana (restorative or rejuvenation) drug. The drug is given in nervine, cardiac, respiratory, urinary, mental, senile, rhaematic reminal and blood pressure complaints.

The drug is considered to possess anti-cancer properties and it has also protective action in particular.

57. Woodfordia Fruiticosa (L.) Kurz. syn. Woodfordia floribunda Salisb.

Lythraceae

Dhātakī (Āyurveda)

Dhai, Dhatki, Dhamai (Hindi/common names)

Large leafy and straggling shrub, with long spreading branches; shrub attaining height upto 6 meters; bark smooth, cinnamon brown. Leaves opposite or in whord of three subsessile, 5-10 cm. long, oblong-lanceolate, round or cordate at the base, entire. Flowers numerous, red in dense, axillary, paniculate clusters, fls. in short cymes. Furit capsular, 1cm. long, usually splitting the calyx near the base, irregularly, enclosed within calyx-tube; seeds many minute. Flowering and fruiting in February-June.

Plant is occuring throughout India particulary in greater part and extending upto 1500 -1600 meters in subtropical and lower temperate regions in Himalayas.

The flowers and plant yeild tannin upto 20 percent.

The flowers are mainly used in medicine. Being a strong astringent and haemostatic herbal agent, the drug is useful in dysentery, diarrhoea, menorrhagia, liver disorders, haemorrhoids, disorders of mucous membrance, leucorrhoea, bowel complaints and other similar diseases. Externally it is used in uncers, chaneres, burn, haemorrhage, sores, cuts injuries and similar conditions as effective healing and blood coogulating remedy good in burns and wounds. Flowers are commonly employed in pharmaceutics as fermentation (alcohol generating) and colouring agent.

The drug is considered to possess anti-cancer activity. Flowers have been reported to be useful in treatment of cancer.

CLASSICAL FORMULATIONS OF AYURVEDA USEFUL IN CANCER

A. RASAYOGA

Formulation	Source
1. Sarveśvara parpaṭ	(Rasaratna samuccaya, vidradhi adhikāra)
2. Bṛhad loknātha rasa	(Bhaisjya ratnāvalī)
3. Gaṇḍamātha rasa	(Auṣadha gunadharma śāstra)
4. Mahālakṣmī vilāsa rasa	Ibid.
5. Rasamāṇikya	
6. Śuddha gandhaka	
7. Gandhaka rasāyana	: Rasmdra sāra sangraha
8. Āditya rasa	
9. Vidyā vāgeṣvarī rasa	Rasacandrikā
10. Rāja tāleśvara rasa	Rasendra sāsa sangraha
11. Roudra rasa	Ibid.
12. Vaḍvānala rasa	Ibid.
13. Ardhanāris rasa	Ibid.
14. Candrakalā rasa	Yogaratnākara
15. Pāśupata rasa	Ibid.
16. Vitaṃḍava rasa	Rasendrasāra samgraha
17. Makaradhvaja	
18. Mallasindūra	Siddhayoga sangraha
19. Tālasindūra	Siddha bhaiṣgymaṇimāla
20. Śilasindūra	Rasendra sāra sangraha
21. Viyādhiharaṇa Rasāyana	Rasendra sāra sangraha
22. Rasakarpūra	
23. Haragvurimalla yoga	
24. Candrāmrta rasa	
25. Sarvasiddha rasāyana	
26. Kāmadudhā rasa	
27. Jayamaṅgala rasa	
28. Viśrambhara rasa	
29. Soumeśvara rasa	

30. Tāleśvara rasa
31. Mahākaleśvara rasa
32. Śitāri rasa
33. Nṛpativallabha rasa
34. Trailokya Cintāmaṇī rasa
35. Lakṣmīnārāyana rasa
36. Arakeśvara rasa
37. Pratāpa lankeśvara rasa
38. Bṛhad lokanātha rasa
39. Amīra rasa
40. Ṣaṇṇmukha rasāyana
41. Tuttha rasāyana
42. Rasasindūra

B. GUGGULU YOGA

1. Pancatikta ghṛta guggulu
2. Kaiśoura guggulu
3. Kāṅcanāra guggulu
4. Paṅcaviṃśati guggulu
5. Triphalā guggulu
6. Mahāyogarāja guggulu
7. Vraṇāri guggulu
8. Gokṣurādi guggulu

C. ĀSAVĀRIṢTA

1. Abhayāriṣta
2. Khadirāriṣṭa
3. Rohitakāriṣṭa
4. Sārivādyāsava
5. Punarna vāriṣṭa
6. Pippdyāsava
7. Bhṛṅgarājājāsava
8. Mṛtasanjī vanī sura
9. Daśamūlāriṣṭa

10. Vāsāriṣṭa
11. Candanāsava
12. Uśīrāsava

D. CŪRṆA

1. Triphalā cūrṇa
2. Copacīnyādi cūrṇa
3. Pancanimba cūrna
4. Maṅjiṣṭhādi cūrṇa
5. Nyagrodhādi cūrna
6. Sitopalādi cūrṇa
7. Vadyabhāskara cūrṇa

E. KVĀTHA

1. Maṅjiṣṭhādi kvātha
2. Bṛhat maṅjiṣṭhādi kvātha
3. Piunarnavāṣṭaka kvātha
4. Varuṇādi kvātha
5. Udumbarādi kvātha
6. Mahārāsnādi kvātha

F. LEPA

1. Daśāṅga lepa
2. Sarṣapādi pralepa

G. BHSSMA - PIṢṬĪ

1. Hīraka bhasma
2. Svarṇa bhasma
3. Abhraka bhasma

   Kānta louha bhasma

5. Tuttha bhasma
6. Vaṅga bhasma
7. Tāmra bhasma
8. Vimalabhasma
9. Nāgabhasma
10. Pancaratnapiṣṭī

11. Mūkta piṣṭī
12. Śveta bhasma
13. Svarṇa mākṣika bhasma
14. Jaharmohara piṣṭī
15. Louha bhasma
16. Muktāpancāmṛta
17. Hiṅgula bhasma
18. Haratāla bhasma
19. Mayūracandrikā bhasma
20. Tāmrabhasma
21. Śankhabhasma

H. ARKA

1. Arbudavāṇa arka

I. TAILA

1. Malla taila
2. Jātyādi taila
3. Karvīrādya taila
4. Candanabalā lakāṣādi taila
5. Yaṣṭimādhvādi taila
6. Ṣaḍabindu taila
7. Amṛtādi taila

J. VAṬĪ

1. Candrapraplehā vaṭī
2. Śilājatvādi vaṭī
3. Ārogyavardhinī vaṭī
4. Rasāñjana ghana vaṭī
5. Sanjīvani vaṭī
6. Śūlavajriṇī vaṭī
7. Punarnovā ghana vaṭī
8. Sudarśana vaṭī
9. Bṛhad śivā guṭikā
10. Yogottama vaṭī
11. Viṣamuṣṭika vaṭī

12. Gajanālakeśvara rasa (vaṭi)

K. RASĀYANA

1. Amṛtabhallātaka rasāyana
2. Madhusnuhī rasāyana

L. SATVA

1. Amṛtā (guḍucī) stava

M. LOUHA-MAṆḌŪRA

1. Punarnavādi maṇḍūra
2. Dhātri louha
3. Navāyasa louha
4. Candanādi louha
5. Ahicandra louha
6. Śilājatvādi louha

N. PARPAṬĪ

1. Vijaya parpaṭī
2. Pancāmṛta parpaṭī
3. Vajra parpaṭī
4. Svarṇaparpaṭī

O. AVALEHA

1. Drākṣāvaleha
2. Vāsavaleha

P. GHṚTA

1. Mahātriphalā ghṛta
2. Brāhmī ghṛta
3. Triphalā ghṛta
4. Mahātriphalādya ghṛta

Q. VARTI

1. Candrodaya varti

APPENDIX

LITERATURE : WHO MATERIAL ON CANCER

A. PUBLICATIONS

1. A Rational approach to Radio-diagnostic Investigations, TRS No. 683, 1983.
2. Assessment of the Carcinogenicity and Mutagenicity of chemicals, TRS No. 546, 1974
3. Bibliography on the Eipdemiology of cancer, 1946-1960, 1983.
4. Cancer Control in children, EURO, R.&S. No. 75, 1983.
5. Cancer Control , TRS No. 251, 1963
6. Cancer pain Relief, 1986.
7. Cancer Statistics, TRs No. 322, 1986
8. Cancer Treatment, TRs No. 322, 1986
9. Cytological Screening in the control of cervical cancers, Technical Guidelines, 1988.
10. Development of cancer centres and community cancer control programmes, EURO R&S No. 70, 1982
11. Drug Therapy of cancer, (Brule, G. etal), 1973
12. Early Detection of Cancer, TRS No. 422, 1969
13. Gestational Trophoplastic Diseases, TRs No. 692, 1983.
14. Guide to short-term Test for Detecting Mutagenic and Carcinogenic Chemicals, ERC No. 51, 1985.
15. Histopathological Definition of Burkitts tumour, 1969
16. Immunotherapy of Cancer, TRS No. 344, 1966
17. Interferon Therapy, TRs No. 676, 1982
18. International Classification of Diseases for Oncology (ICD.O), 1976.
19. Optimization of Radiotherapy, particularly in Developing Countries, TRs No. 644, 1980.
20. Prevention of Cancer, TRs No. 276, 1964.

21. Principles for the Testing and Evaluation of Drugs for Carcinogenecity, TRs No. 426, 1969.
22. Steroid contraception and the Risk of Neoplasia, TRS No. 619, 1978.
23. Trends in Cancer Research, 1966.
24. Viruses and Cancer, TRS No. 295, 1965.
25. WHO handbook for reporting results of cancer treatment, offset Pub No. 48, 1976.
26. WHO handnbook for standardised cancer registries (Hospital based), offeset Pub. No. 25, 1976.
27. Prevention of Liver Cancer, TRS No. 691, 1983.
28. Cancer in costa Rica, ARC, TR No. 1, 1988.

    [source : WHO publications : 1947-1988; Catalogue October 1988; SEA, pp. 4-5, 78-79, 127-129,

B. IIARC (International Agency for Research on Cancer) Publication,

IARC Annual Reports, IARC Monographs on the Evaluation of careinogenic Risk of Chemicals to Humans and the IARC Information Bulletin on the Survey of chemicals being tested for carcinogenicity: Several volumes and supplements.

C. IHCT (International Histological Classification of Tumours) comprises a series of works (illustrated by colour photographs and transparencies), giving definitions, classifications and nomenclatures of cancer types, based on internationally agreed histological criteria Acceptable alike to physicians, surgeons, radiologists, pathologists, and statisticians, the classification facilities collaboration among cancer workers throughout the world and provides a series of invaluable treaching instruments. Some important works in the series (1 to 26) follow :

1. Histological Typing of Lung Tumours.
2. Histological Typing of Breast Tumours.
5. Histological Typing of Odontogenic Tumours
6. Histological Typing of Bone Tumours
7. Histological Typing of Salivary Gland Tumours
8. Cytology of the Female Genital Tract (Riotton, G. et al)
9. Histological Typing of Ovarian Tumours

10. Histological Typing of Urinary Bladder Tumours
11. Histological Typing of Thyroid Tumours (Hedinger, C. et al)
12. Histological Typing of Skin Tumours (Ten Seldam, R.F.J. et al)
13. Histological Typing of Female Genital Tract Tumours (Poulsun, H.E. etal)
14. Histopathological and Cytological Typing of Neoplastic Diseases of haematopoietic and Lymphoid tissues (Mathe, G. et al)
15. Histological Typing of Intestinal Tumours (marron, B.C. et al)
16. Histological Typing of Testis Tumours (Mostofi, F.K. et al)
17. Cytology of Non-gynaecological sites (Riotton, G. et al)
18. Histological Typing of Gastric and Oesophageal Tumours (Qota, K. et al)
19. Histological Typing of Upper Respiratory Tract Tumours (Shanmungratnam, K. et al)
20. Histological Typing of Tumours of the Liver, Biliary Tract and Pancreas (Gibson, J.B. et al)
21. Histological Typing of tumours of Central Nervous System (Zulch, K.J. et al)
22. Histological Typing of Prostate tumours (Mostofi, F.K. et al)
23. Histological Typing of Endocrine tumours (Williams, E.D. et al)
24. Histological Typing of tumours of the Eye and its Adnexa (Zimmerman, L.E.)
25. Histological Typing of Kidney tumours (Mostofi, f.K. et al)
26. A coded compendium of the International Histological Classification of Tumours (sobin, L.H. et al)

SELECTED BIBLIOGRAPHY

A. Caraka Saṃhitā

Suśruta Saṃhitā

Aṣṭāṅga Sangraha

Aṣṭāṅga Hṛdaya

Mādhava Nidāna

Śāraṅgadhara Saṃhitā

Rasendrasāra Sangraha

Rasaratna Samuccaya

Rasatantrasāra va Siddha Yogasangraha

Rasataraṅginī

Rasajalanidhi

Rasaprakaśa Sudhākara

Rasayoga Sāgara

Rasendra Cuṇāmaṇi

Rasārṇava

Rasaratnākara

Rasahṛdayatandra

Rasakāmadhenu

Rasaprakaśa Sudhākara

Rasāmṛta

Bhaiṣajya Ratnāvalī

Yogaramākara

Gadanigraha

Vasavarājī yam
Yogacintamaṇi
Bhāvaprakāśa
Arkaprakāśa
Vaidya yoga ratnāvalī
Vaidyajīvanama

Siddha Bhaiṣajya Maṇimālā
Siddhayoga Sangraha
Siddha prayoga latikā
Au]sadha gu]nadharma «s"astra
Cakradatta
Vangasena
Ayurveda Prakāśaa
Vṛndamādhava
Vaidyamanoramā
Kalyāṇakāraka
Sahasrayoga
Ānandakandam

Dhamvantari Nighaṇṭu
Rāja Nighaṇṭu
Kaiyadeva Nighaṇṭu
Bhāvaprakāśa Nighaṇṭu
Soḍhala Nighantu
Vanouṣadhi Candrodaya
Madanapāla Nighantu
Bṛhannighaṇṭuratnākara

B. Hooker, J.D. — Flora of British India, Vols. 1-7, London, 1872-1897

Anonymous — Wealth of India (Raw Materials), vols. 1-8, CSIR, New Delhi, 1986-69.

Anonymous : Medicinal Plants of India, Vol. I, ICMR, New Delhi, 1967.

Anonymous : The Ayurvedic formulary of India, Part I & II, govt. of India, Ministry of Health & F.W., New Delhi, 1978, 1990s.

Chopra, R.N. et al : Glossary of Indian Medicinal Plants, CSIR, New Delhi, 1956.

: Supplement to Glossary of Indian Medicinal Plants, CSIR, New Delhi, 1969.

: Second Supplement to G.I.M.P., Part I, CSIR, New Delhi, 1992.

: Indigenous Drugs of India, 2nd. Ed., Calcutta, 1958.

Jain, S.K. : Dictionary of Indian Folk Medicine and Ethnobotany, New Delhi, 1991.

Kirtikar, K.R. et al : Indian Medicinal Plants, Vols. 1-4, allahabad, 1953.

Mukerji, B : Indian Pharmaceutical codex, CSIR, Vol.I, New Delhi, 1953.

Nadkarni, K.M. : Indian Materia Medica, 2nd Vol., 3rd Ed., Bombay, 1954.

Pandey, Gyanendra : Vanoussạdhi Mañjuṣā (Useful Medicinal Plants of the plains), by Prof. Ram Nath Vaidya, Hardwar, 1990.

: Medicinal Flowers - Puṣpāyurveda

: Medicinal Flowers of India and Adjascent Regions, Delhi, 1992.

: Gyanendra Enumeratio Plantamedica - Gyanendra Auṣadhīya Pādaāvali (Edited by Sumitra Pandey), Delhi, 1993.

: Uncommon Plant Drugs of Ayurveda (Section I-III), Delhi, 1993.

: Ayurvedic Cikitsā Kośa, Delhi, 1995.

: Medicinal Plants of Himalaya, Vol. I (Illustrated), Delhi, 1995.

: Some Lesser Known Herbal Drugs in Ayurveda, Delhi, 1996.

: Traditional Medicine in South-East Asia and Indian Medical Science, Delhi, 1997.

: Puṣpam Samarpayāmi - Bhāratiya Sanskriti me Vanaspatiyan, Delhi, 1997.

: Camatkari Jadibutiyan, Delhi, 1998.

: System of Plant Nomenclature in Āyurveda, Varanasi, 1997.

: Uttarakhanda Ki Vanouṣadhiyān, Varanasi, 1999.

: Medicinal Plants of Himalaya, Vol. II, Delhi, 1999.

: Dravyaguṇa Vijnāna (English-Sanskrit), Vol. I, 1998; Vol. II, 2001; Varanasi; and Vol III (under publication).

Sharma, P.V. : Dravyaguna Vigyan, Part II, Varanasi, 1956.

Singh, D. : Yunani Dravyaguna, Part III, Lucknow, 1978.

Taber, C.W. : Cyclopedic Medical Dictionary, Philadelphia, 1960.

Vaidya, B.G. : Nighantu Adarsha, Vol. I-II, Varanasi, 1965-68.

In addition, various journals / periodicals / reports / seminar abstracts related to different aspects of diseases, management and drugs as well as modern literature on oncology/cancerology and allied subjects/aspects.

PLANT NAMES (BOTANICAL)

DRUGS NAMES (AYURVEDA)